The Health Bible

Rob Sutton

Distributed by
Optymal Health Studios Corporation
185 Brock Street North, Unit 1
Whitby, ON
L1N-4H3
Tel. (905) 556-2202
Email: rob@optymalhealthstudios.com

www.optymalhealthstudios.com
www.canadianhealthbible.com

ISBN-13: 978-1494386573
ISBN-10: 1494386577

The information provided in this book is designed to provide helpful information on the subjects discussed. This book is not meant to be used, nor should it be used, to diagnose or treat any medical condition. For diagnosis or treatment of any medical problem, consult your own physician. The publisher and author are not responsible for any specific health or allergy needs that may require medical supervision and are not liable for any damages or negative consequences from any treatment, action, application or preparation, to any person reading or following the information in this book. References are provided for informational purposes only and do not constitute endorsement of any websites or other sources. Readers should be aware that the websites listed in this book may change.

Editor: Suzan Burpee and Amanda Denmans
Cover Design: Jesse Messenger
Written in Canada Baby! Woo!

REAL HEALTH BIBLE
TESTIMONIALS

I want to thank you for the help, support, and training you have given me. You have helped me achieve my goal of losing 50lbs and more. I am truly grateful for being a part of such a wonderful family. Thank you!
– **Moreen R.**

I was suffering from a shoulder injury and was experiencing exercise-induced tension headaches which made working out both challenging and painful. Training has helped me to not only eliminate my exercise related pain, but meet my goals as well. I can now exercise pain-free and look and feel great!
– **Elise F.**

I never thought I would be able to do such workouts! Thank you for giving me the opportunity to prove to myself that I could and for seeing the potential in me. You were essential in pushing me through my weaknesses and praising my strengths.
– **Suzanne L.**

It's amazing how my life has changed! I have done a complete 180 in terms of my health and my personality. I feel like I can take on the world! Never in my life have I had a group of people believe in me like this. Your kindness and care has changed my life forever. You have given me so much I cannot express it!
– **Yvonne R.**

"This has changed my family's lives! I knew exercise and proper nutrition was the answer, but could not find the time and I was too lazy to make it. I am 45 years of age and feel and look better than I ever have. Fitness and nutrition have become a way of life for my kids and me. Thank you for all your help, guidance, and hard work."
– Kim B.

"You need to take care of your body; it's the only place you have to live." My goal now is to inspire and to be inspired by everyone I meet. That's what Optimal Health is all about. My recipe for success is inspiration, determination, and a positive attitude."
– Tanya B.

"My day to day energy has improved and I am now able to create my own workout plans and continue to work out multiple times a week on my own. This program taught me everything I know about healthy eating from what to buy at the grocery store to how to make fresh healthy juices."
– Stephan B.

"This has given me the tools to stay successful in my quest. It has helped me learn new things I would have never related to my own personal fitness and lifestyle. Most of all, Rob has made my journey incredibly fun and his ability to motivate people is unparalleled to anyone I have ever met before."
– Mark K.

CONTENTS

1   The Bigger Picture   1

2   Health Illiterate   3

3   Junk Food Junkie to Health Club Owner   5

4   Widespread Confusion   13

5   Frequently Asked Questions   25

6   Take A Brain Dump   32

7   The 10 Health Commandments   37

8   The Ultimate Body Transformation Secret   64

9   Detox & Dietary Guide   72

10 Eat Clean & Train Dirty   89

11 Scientific Fat Loss   129

12 Saving Time & Money   140

13 Mentally & Physically Fit   162

14 Focus On Health Not Wealth   178

    About The Author

    Field Notes

    My Gift To You ;)

THE TEN HEALTH COMMANDMENTS

Live One Meal At A Time - Eat Every 2-3 Hours

First Things First - Get Alkaline

Progress, Not Perfection - Eat Protein Every Meal

Sweat Everyday - Carbs Are Exercise Earned

Fat Is Not Evil – Supplement Healthy Oils

Keep It Simple - Carry A Water Bottle Everywhere

Don't Fail To Plan - Prep Your Food Before

Early To Bed, Early To Rise - Eat Smaller Meals

Get Grounded – Shop At The Farmers' Market

Live And Let Live - Plan Your Cheat Meals

1
THE BIGGER PICTURE

Albert Einstein once said, "we can't solve problems with the same thinking that we created them with." When I was younger my parents always told me to keep an open mind, and look into things a little more before accepting them as fact. You have to be willing to look past conventional thinking for alternative viewpoints. Don't be afraid of going back and starting from the beginning, you may be surprised to see where it leads you. Using The Health Bible will require you to take some notes and do some field testing to find out what works best for you. I did mine through my travels by experiencing all kinds of different cultures and comparing their belief systems to new research studies shown to me by the "experts."

Very rarely have I seen a person fail who has thoroughly followed this path. Those that don't find themselves in the best shape of their life, are people who cannot, or will not completely give themselves to this simple program. The key word to understand here is completely! It's critical in the beginning for you to be truly honest with yourself about your situation, and what you can do to improve it. Sometimes this can be hard for us to do, and you're not at fault! Sometimes we can be running around on autopilot so fast, that it becomes difficult to grasp and develop a new way of daily living that demands rigorous honesty. Without this your chances are less than average. There are those, too, who suffer from serious mental and physical health disorders, but many of us do improve if we have the capacity to be honest about our diet and lifestyle choices.

If you can disclose in a general way what you used to be like, what happened, and what you are like now, then you are ready for The Health Bible and the steps it suggests. If you have decided what you want and are willing to go to any length to get it, then you can take on "The Ten Health Commandments" as a suggested program of improvement. At some of these steps you may hesitate. Or maybe you could find an easier, softer way. I assure you there isn't one! With all the willingness that you can find, I beg of you to be fearless and thorough from the very start. Half measures will availed you nothing! Some of us tried to hold on to our old ideas and the result was nil until we let go completely.

2

HEALTH ILLITERATE

I was fired from every job I ever had…until I started working at a gym. After years working in the nutrition and fitness industry, spending thousands of dollars on personal training, opening my own facilities and trying everything possible to look the way I wanted to look, I realized something was missing. I had a huge problem on my hands! If I, as a personal trainer, was finding it hard to pull myself together, what the hell was the average person going through?

Looking for options, I noticed there was a huge industry separation between nutrition and fitness and most people were following advice that was just not good for them. It's usually one or the other: you either eat clean and don't work out, or you stuff garbage in your face and only hit the gym every few days.

There are literally thousands of so called nutrition and fitness "experts" out there pushing all kinds of pills, bars, shakes, and snake oil remedies to help you lose the extra pounds. The truth is, it's hard to find educated, nonbiased advice! This is because the people that are truly leading the research are stuck in a lab finding out amazing and useful information that is then reported to multinational health organizations. These organizations then produce information that's diverged so much from the original information, due to both outside factors and personal agendas, that it ends up screwing us all up. From that alone, we have created an overabundance of health experts offering advice on diet and exercise. In addition, these experts keep their information and advice overly complex so their customers will feel their "secret" is worth way more than it actually is.

Just take a minute to think about where you found this book. If you're sitting in the book section right now, you probably had about 500 other choices on the shelf. I think keeping things unnecessarily confusing by having plans that are too ridged or plans that are dependent on too many factors, is a big problem, so I'm taking care of that right now. I wrote this book to clarify and educate the average person on scientifically rigorous nutrition and fitness information.

Personally, I think it's not too late to turn around the massive epidemic of diabetic and obese children being outlived by their parents. The statistics on this one don't lie! By simply clarifying and educating, I hope to change the lives of parents and their children. I can personally guarantee you may know someone that could definitely benefit from reading this. You can be sure they'll personally thank you for changing their outlook on everything.

3

JUNK FOOD JUNKIE
TO HEALTH CLUB OWNER

You could say I got my education from the school of hard knocks. I've lived all over the world and it all started when I failed 9th grade French. I decided to make up my credit by doing an exchange to France. When I came back, I noticed that things are very different outside of North America. What I've attributed to this experience is how important it is to get outside your comfort zone and see how other people are living in other parts of the world. If you haven't done that yet, I recommend putting this book down right now and planning a trip. Don't think or look at hotels, just do it! You can figure out places to stay when you arrive. While I wouldn't recommend an all-inclusive down south, if you do settle for that, at least bring this book with you. It's good to remember to stay open-minded to other things, cultures, and tricks if you want to improve your health on a daily basis. I caught the "Travel Bug" and opted for more life experience instead of going back to school and racking up debt. As an expatriate, I was exposed to the eastern philosophies of medicine such as martial arts, reflexology, acupuncture, and Reiki; all things that Western society views as alternative therapies or Chinese voodoo fairy magic. Now that sounds interesting! But let's be serious.

I come from a very good family and always knew the difference between right and wrong. The thing was, I was too young and selfish to care. There was no way I could have seen the problems I was about to face as a result of my actions. Less than three years ago, I had no job, no money, no license, no direction, and no real friends. I had a college education in a field I didn't like and a whole lot of experience failing at great opportunities – and about $16 to my name. I could essentially tell you two stories at this point. As time goes on it became clearer to me when one story began to proceed the other. I could let you know that I have lived all over the world leveraging amazing opportunities, or I could be honest and mention that I was trying to run away from my deepest shortcomings, instead of actually facing them.

I got the travel bug pretty early in life. Failing grade nine French, I decided to make up some credits by packing everything into my snowboard bag and attending school in Grenoble France. This was a dream come true! What high school kid doesn't want to hit double black diamond runs three days a week? Becoming a ski bum, I got incredibly good at boarding, but I wasn't that excited about going to school from eight to six. It's funny because in school I was always labeled dyslexic, but most of the world's languages are spoken or interpreted backwards. The problem wasn't that my brain was reversing things, it was that English is an inferior language and they were trying to impose on me. Needless to say I made friends, learned French fast, and managed to acquire quality Cognac Liquor every day, instead of going to class. I knew what I was doing wasn't healthy, but it seemed to be a lot easier to make friends and fit in this way considering the language barrier. I was young, dumb, and full of Rum, avoiding hard work and focus anyway I could.

High school finished… I was off to attend the only college program that accepted me. My bad habits lead to more missed classes and a lot of good times that shaped my personality into what it is today. The "Jimi Hendrix" lifestyle was extremely contradictory to the Police Foundations diploma I was half-heartedly striving for. This particular area of my life could easily be a book all in its own. All of my social tsunamis and quasi-criminal activity left me with some skills that were transferable, if I could find my passion.

After graduation, I decided to build some life experience and move to Shanghai. I found a martial arts school close to my flat and jumped into every type of Kung-Fu I could find. This was my first introduction to the Eastern philosophy of culture and medicine. I was smiling every day. This is when my partying began to peak for the worst, and when I really started to try hard to make things work. It's ironic to think that although I drank and partied for years trying to get the world-class job, car and girlfriend I wanted, it wasn't until I stopped all this that I actually got any of those things. I started taking Mandarin lessons every day to give myself the feeling that I was "going back to school again." I learned a lot from this and I believe it allowed me to access parts of my brain that I'd never used before. Mandarin is a pictorial language, which means they use symbols to communicate meaning. I think this is a much better way to communicate and that alone changed my perception forever.

With deteriorating health and lack of sobriety, I decided to move on again and re-locate to Prague where I could easily find an English teaching job and continue my Hendrix lifestyle in the club scene and local breweries. I was evicted from two flats in my first two months and couldn't stop losing the little things like my wallet and shoes every other day. I got sick of not holding down a job, having no money and only eating potatoes with no place to stay. I got a return ticket home feeling ten times lower then when I left.

I hit rock bottom. Over the past five years, my evolution from Jersey Shore party animal to health club owner was so fast, no one knew who I was anymore. A few years ago, I moved to Toronto in hopes to make something of myself. I obtained a job at a large gym cleaning up the weights and handling customer service with the members on the floor. This was the beginning of my career in the fitness industry. I watched all the trainers closely and asked so many questions that I became known as Random Robby.

My thoughts were going a million miles a minute and I finally felt like I actually fit in. This environment was so conducive to my so-called Attention Deficit Disorder (A.D.D.) that I managed to naturally turn myself into an asset for the company. If there is one thing I have learned from this experience, it's that the quality and quantity of questions you ask is directly related to your success. They may not be the best quality questions, but the quantity was there and sometimes I'm more balls then brains. I knew I was lacking in my knowledge of nutrition, so I capitalized on my position and negotiated a deal with the best trainer they had. I asked him if he would trade me some referrals from my chats with members on the floor, in exchange for some free sessions. This was my first experience with a personal trainer and, if you haven't worked with one before, I highly recommend that you put it on your bucket list.

Shortly thereafter, a sales position came up and I didn't even think twice about accepting it. I was in heaven, but, it turned out that sales wasn't enough for me. I wanted to be on the floor with the trainers, learning how to better myself and how to help others do the same. The commission had me making more money than ever before and I was finally able to afford a few more sessions with my trainer. I knew I wanted to learn everything he knew, so I offered myself as a "guinea pig" for some of the new systems he was developing on nutrition and fitness. Once I started to get more time and experience under my belt, my strategy was simple: spend hours on the floor talking about everything I was learning, so that when the time came to get certified it wouldn't be a problem.

After a month, the roles reversed from me learning from members, to me teaching the members. I even started filling up nutrition seminars for my trainer. We became partners in crime and this really was the happiest I had ever been. He taught me that once you get in the best shape of your life, your insurance policy was to help others to the same thing. I started getting involved with all kinds of new things from juice cleansing experiments to a 600km bike rally from Toronto to Montreal, and even traveling with clients to Europe for some perogies.

My second client, who I had been working with for a few months, lost any progress we gained every time he traveled on business. So, he asked me to go with him! We were gone for two weeks, and he handled the expenses. This was a challenge because my program design had to include working with no equipment, and it had to be enjoyable and flexible for any circumstances. I don't know if you've ever been to Poland in the winter, but they love to eat and drink. This was not just a professional struggle, but a personal one because those two weeks were a reminder of my old lifestyle that I left behind in the not-so-distant past. Every morning I had to check myself into the role I was playing as a trainer, while my old self was constantly trying to draw me back into the darkness. By day four I had accumulated so much emotional struggle, I was in tears. My only option was to wipe my eyes and put on the biggest smile I could muster. I had remembered a quote by Tony Robbins, "changing your physiology will change your psychology." It all started with forced smiles and emotional anguish, but it lead to an active, healthy lifestyle. I found my "medicine", and it was my responsibility to share it with the world.

Shortly thereafter, I realized my love for fitness expanded beyond the corporate company I was representing, so I took the leap of faith and started my own gym. As you can imagine, it's scary starting an entirely new, demanding business venture when you can hardly even buy your own groceries. I wrote my business plan, received some government grants, and got busy. With all the risk I had taken on, the responsibilities began to mount.

Now, these were good responsibilities, but responsibilities nonetheless. I ended up doing most of the renovations myself and sleeping at my soon-to-be gym for a few months. After the renovations were complete, Optymal Health Studios finally opened! I learned very quickly that an area I had to focus on was time management. Time is the most valuable asset we have. Having a complete juice bar in the gym brought in a lot of people in but it left me with no free time. This lead me to the next step in my business adventure: hiring staff. I wasn't making any money, initially, however I had my business plan to follow. These struggles were very real, but I made it through them. My dream became a reality in Optymal Health Studios. I didn't let anything hold me back from succeeding. It was one interesting year that was huge for personal growth. I bit the bullet, took the risk, and kept the faith as I walked the path from junk food junkie to health club owner, and into The Health Bible.

With this book, I wanted to give you everything that I found to work for myself and all of my clients. Interestingly enough, I feel I learn more about myself from listening to other people's problems. I still have more to learn and I am relatively young, but I respect anyone who has more years in the game of life than me because they've had more life experiences. I've found the mistakes we make teach us way more about ourselves than our "homerun hits," and if we can share our mistakes, we can get through them easier. A problem shared is a problem halved!

There might be a lot of bad information on nutrition and fitness out there, but the reality is this: taking a risk and trying something new is much more powerful than spending months trying to figure out what to do. Just take action and do something! We seem to have lost our way by over-complicating things. Often, I find myself going back to the things my grandparents used to say. Some of that ancient wisdom does have good information hidden within it. All it can take sometimes is a short one-liner like "eat your veggies" to completely change your outlook. If you make it easier to read or listen to, it's memorable! You'll soon see I am not short on any one liners. Humility aside, I have made every mistake there is to make in the field of diet and exercise and that's why I do what I do. My story really is a rags-to-riches kind of thing, just without the riches - yet. To be honest, the more I learn about what's important in life, the more I prefer to live like Ghandi, with very few worldly possessions. He was able to find everything he desired in his passions. I've found my true passion in helping big people make big changes.

I was once asked, "If you were to die and leave everyone with one secret, what would it be?" I thought about what caused me to go from Joe Schmo trainer to health club owner, and above all else, it was writing down my goals. I'm not talking about just thinking about them, actually writing them down! Keeping things in the realm of contemplation is useless. You keep thinking about the same things over and over again instead of expanding on that thought – and taking action. Look at it this way, you probably have 4 or 5 things that you really think about over the course of the day, and we rarely ever figure them out. We just think about the same things again and again. Improper action is better than no action at all.

4

WIDESPREAD CONFUSION

People just don't know where to start! You need confidence when it comes to what you put in your body and when you exercise. From what I've found, the easiest way to remember information is to stick some humor into it and make a positive emotional connection.

It's very easy to get bogged down with diet information and get "analysis paralysis." That's the real problem we all face: we make excuses for not taking action. Think of our behavior like a record player playing music. If you look closely at the record, you'll see very small patterns that the needle runs along creating the unique sounds you hear. These "music patterns" reflect patterns in our behavior. Over the years I've developed different ways to scratch out these small patterns that are not conducive to health and wellness. Think of them as "thought-starters" and "thought-stoppers." If we can start changing the small stuff, like taking a different way to work, packing our lunch, or not starting the day with a donut, then we will begin to change the bigger picture, or the over-all sound of our music. We are creatures of habit and usually, our habits suck.

When you are dealing with diet and exercise, you're dealing with habits and behavior. When you're dealing with habit-based behavior, you're dealing with time management. The habits you have throughout the day are directly connected to your eating and exercise patterns. It's important you have a good grasp on how you're going to start to change those patterns of behavior. This is about dealing with the psychology of you as a unique person. You need strategies designed specifically around educating yourself so those choices get easier and easier. Each day should get better, if you're diligent. A really good coach/teacher/trainer/program/book should act as a constructive feedback system that provides you with information on the things you're doing that you may not even be aware of.

Currently, we are dealing with a massive public health problem that costs us billions of dollars annually, shortens the lives of our children, and causes the general public to suffer many different illnesses. Rates of obesity have almost doubled in the last 25 years, yet studies suggest we are not eating more food, nor eating more fat or exercising less, to account for this crisis. With the increase in convenience stores and T.V. dinners, our food culture has been transformed. We are swimming in sugars. Refined white sugar, high fructose corn syrup, dextrose, maltose, lactose, sorbitol, and xylitol (to name a few), are all different kinds of sugars. They are the major ingredients in almost all processed foods, from canned goods to cereal. Bookmark this page and take a quick look around your kitchen for these little devils. They're hidden in plain sight. Additional forms of sugars are not the only problem. Any "starchy" carbohydrates we consume such as pasta, white flour breads, chips and snacks might as well be sugar. Sugar is a food uniquely designed to turn into fat. Within minutes of entering the body, carbohydrates metabolize and actually rob other vital nutrients from the body so it can be processed, further depleting your system. The havoc these sugars and flavoring chemicals wreak on the hormonal system adds another huge dynamic to the problem.

As a result of these highly-processed foods with fake sugars and hidden chemicals, our healthcare system is overburdened! Disease counts are higher than ever and the problem only gets worse. Once a diagnosis is made, the average person looks to the healthcare system for a cure and usually ends up with medication. However, effectively combating things like obesity and working to prevent disease requires much more than bottles of pills. It requires a fundamental shift in food choices and increased physical activity. With rapidly-increasing healthcare costs, society is welcoming all natural and holistic products like this book. Responsibility is finally being placed back onto the individual to treat the cause – not just the symptom.

Think back to your childhood relationship with food, did you grow up on processed junk food? Were pizza and hotdogs the average meal for yourself and your peers at school? For some reason, my principals and parents thought that junk was okay to feed the future generations. With this sort of relationship with food, and not much exercise, it's only a matter of time until you're diagnosed with A.D.D. as I was. Surely an introduction to the western philosophy of medicine could help!

Your mental and emotional states are a direct correlation to your diet. It's no wonder I couldn't focus! I was operating on sugar, margarine and whatever food dyes were in the "food" I ate. In fact, all of these early-life experiences created the majority of problems I faced over the years.

In high school, I started working out a bit, but I never touched any "good" foods. After I graduated and went to college, I continued to run from my problems and, in-turn, caused more with the same-old habits. Then I started working at a gym when it finally hit me: my dietary control was non-existent! I was so caught up in counting calories, that I had my first trainer make me a menu plan centred solely on pizza and chocolate milk. It's funny how long these food habits can stay with you. Even my ex-girlfriend, who's a die-hard holistic nutritionist, will find herself begging for a McDonald's ice cream (though personally, I prefer Dairy Queen.) Fast food joints are lit up like Disney World, covered in bright siding and sometimes have not one, but two drive-thrus leaving you with a temporary feeling of being satisfied. To add to the effect, they'll send you off with a warm smile and friendly wave – making sure you'll come back soon. Plain and simple: humans are naturally lazy and resistant to change. Especially when every flavor, smell and experience society throws at us is fast, new, and sweeter than high fructose corn syrup.

I decided something had to be done about it. I started making some moves to help solve the problem and have spent a significant amount of time going to schools and businesses discussing how bad the fast and dirty foods are, while generating awareness about the severity of the problem. The root of this issue is convenience (time) and most likely your belief system regarding the last piece of advice on diet you received.

From what I've seen so far in life, there are three things people find difficult to talk about, religion, politics, and nutrition. All of these are based on belief systems, and, when challenged, invoke a passionate response. Even though facts may tell the person otherwise, they rarely waiver from their belief system. During my travels, I began to take notes of different believe systems, with the goal to give the average person a chance to understand proper diet in a no "one-size-fits-all" approach. The Health Bible is a compilation of all the mistakes I've made, and the best advice I could find. I've used it all myself and with hundreds of others to go from Big Mac to six pack. It takes into account all the important factors like age, body type and fitness goals. I wanted to give you full access to all the necessary information while still giving you as much independent decision-making ability as possible. I feel this method is far superior to all "fad diets" because it puts your confidence first, and then gets you to take bigger steps like learning to exercise. Not to mention, I have learned a lot of "ninja tricks," like juice cleansing, which, when done properly, can typically help you lose a healthy 7-14lbs of body fat in very little time.

Most information regarding diets are emotionally charged, often leaving you with negative emotions. My philosophy: emotions destroy intelligence! Don't let that irrational behavior creep into your diet building strategy. For starters, I think you should consider building a basic relationship with your food, then individualize and build off that foundation. Go on a few dates with your diet, take it to second base! Play the field! Try new things! Making compromises if needed, and pencil quality time into your busy schedule.

New smartphone apps, cool websites and infographs are changing the way we learn and absorb information. They appeal to every age group and it's definitely something you'll be seeing more and more on the internet, in books, and in magazines. Many of these new ways of delivering information are helpful simply because of the way that the information is being presented. However, most of the time this information is misinterpreted or simply incorrect.

Infographs are one of my favorite ways of injecting facts into someone's brain. Basically, they're pictures and charts in a comic book-like layout of information. More and more, these are popping up because of how easy it is to get the point across to a large group of people. Just be aware that not everything you read or see is actual fact.

One of my all-time favorite websites that I use regularly is www.StumbleUpon.com. Create an account, check off your interests like nutrition, and start stumbling through info and videos from around the web. It goes along with a philosophy I've always believed in: every now and then, just leave it to chance. The most helpful information I've come across presented itself when I wasn't looking for anything specific. Don't let this add to your confusion though. Remember that anyone can add any website to this so while interesting and thought provoking you should definitely take what you read with a grain of salt.

The internet is definitely a great place to look for

interesting information and keeps the brain juices flowing. This being said, I would not recommend using the internet to self-diagnose any problems. It's likely to be incorrect and will result in you potentially getting all worked up about something you don't need to lose sleep over.

Do a Google search on healthy eating and you'll see there are thousands of contradictory messages from reputable sources. If you're looking for a recipe for success, take everything you read and hear with a grain of salt. The result of good nutrition and fitness combined will have a greater impact than individually. This is a fact we can all agree on. . For example, with a good exercise program, you can lose 1lb a week. With a great nutrition program, you can lose 2lbs a week. Now here's the kicker: with a personalized program combining both nutrition and fitness, it's possible to drop over 3lbs a week on a consistent basis, depending on where you're starting from. This combination has worked for me and can be a very powerful tool. It's a waste of time to try to lose weight with either method alone.

People die every year from compilations directly related to their diet and bad lifestyle choices they are probably not even aware of. If you do the math, hundreds of thousands of people will parish over the next ten years, most from preventable causes. Sadly, unless we experience firsthand, we usually don't seem to grasp the real threat to ourselves and society as a whole.

All of the wide-spread confusion and lack of real understanding regarding what and how much to eat, comes from medical entertainment shows, superficial news coverage, and personal opinions delivered as fact. The Health Bible is my attempt at educating you so you can make an informed decision for yourself. If you want to understand real health and fitness, you should understand the differences between them first. Being fit means you can go out and hit a few volleyballs without needing a defibrillator. I know a lot of people that look great, but are not healthy on the inside. In addition, being healthy isn't just about being disease free. A lot of people have no disease, but they never get any sleep, they have to see their chiropractor every other week, or have to take anti-inflammatories and antihistamines every day.

Opening a health club was relatively easy compared to what I had to face in the years moving forward. Keeping myself on track as well as helping others pull it together, I was up against a highly educated line of human bio chemists and exercise scientist, representing information that went against what I knew worked for me and countless others.

Using The Health Bible will require you look past conventional thinking, to think outside the box and to not be afraid of starting and then re-starting and then re-starting again if it's needed. Find out what works best for you. If it's not working start again and try something new, you never know where it might take you!

So where do we start? Most smooth talking food and fitness experts will hate me for saying this, but start with some mainstream reputable sources of information including Canada's Food Guide, the American Food Pyramid, some university studies and the World Health Organization. I have done a lot of research here and the scientists had their heart in the right place when they came up with these. Whether or not the information is specifically good for you and your situation, is a completely different story. Moving forward, here's the bottom line: 70% of any health and fitness results you are looking to achieve comes from nutrition, 20% come from exercise, and 10% are genetic.

You already know that if you over eat, you'll gain weight! However, what you don't realize that if you under-eat, your body will store every gram of fat and energy you ingest because your body thinks your living through a famine. What are we taught to do? Count calories! Essentially, what ends up happening with this method is that you are always aiming for one target number, but usually hit below more frequently then over. Thus, you're under-eating and keeping your body fat levels the same and your metabolism low.

A more effective get started method if you're counting calories is to use an old martial arts trick I learned from my days living in China: the Universal Law of Averages. This is where a person eats 200 calories over their goal one day, and 200 calories below the next. This factors in most activity levels and hits your target on average more often over the course of a month. It's like aiming for the green, as opposed to shooting for a hole-in-one. You'll hit your mark more often using this method.

The Health Bible principles utilize methods like this with an emphasis on keeping it simple. By not micromanaging your calorie intake, and instead combining the right types of nutrients (at the right times), you'll achieve better results in the long-run. If you start taking out junk snacks and start eating better, you'll probably be under-eating.

Thus, you're not changing your physique that much - if at all! This is why real, lasting results can be so difficult to achieve. The lack of basic understanding can go on and on endlessly. Ask yourself, "Where are my calories coming from? Sugars or starches?" Are you familiar with what carbohydrates are? Generally speaking, your average person does not know that fruits and vegetables are an amazing source of carbohydrates. We are trained to think that carbs are bad for us and that they need to be limited. What you don't realize is that our brain needs at least 132 grams of healthy carbohydrates just for normal brain function. These good carbs are ones we should be getting from fresh fruits and vegetables.

When you remove bad food choices from your diet, you are left with a deficit that you'll need to make up for by eating carbs from healthy sources. The easiest way to get most of your daily value is through juicing. You can either eat 8 (or more) servings of vegetables and fruit, or condense it down by juicing it to make it easier to handle. This is where juice cleansing plays a huge part in a balanced and healthy lifestyle. There are two major benefits to having a juice every day or even taking a 4 to 7 day juice cleanse a few times a year. They detox your body and they help you get alkaline! If you're looking for some direction in this department, you can always check out our websites for more information, or feel free to shoot me an email to rob@optymalhealthstudios.com, and just keep reading on.

It seems when looking for nutrition and fitness guidance, there's a large dividing line between the two. Diet centres generally offer a "one-size-fits-all" approach that involves no quality exercises or motivation to help you along.

Whereas mainstream gyms will make you a personalized fitness program (usually bodybuilding exercises) that barely touch on the more important factor: nutrition! These industries make really good money because people are looking for instant gratification and immediate results. What everyone fails to understand is that almost every body-sculpting process takes at least 6 weeks to get results. Leaving them bored, and frustrated causing them to just drop out of the program.

The truth is, most gyms oversell their memberships and count on you giving up – but still paying to use their stuff. Think of it this way: if you really want to make a lifestyle change that lasts for the rest of your life, take your time and enjoy the process. Don't rush it, and stop paying for memberships you're not using.

Changing behaviours and bad habits can often be the hardest part of the journey. It takes at least 21 days to create a new habit and at least 6 months for it to be fully solidified as a part of our everyday life. We make mistakes, but it's learning from those mistakes that helps us move forward to achieve lasting, long-term results. The most important thing is to learn who your nutritional friends and foes are and address your limiting factors on a day-to-day basis.

If you're looking for help, you'll find that most nutrition and fitness experts will micromanage your program which can consume much of their time and yours. With every client I work with, I identify the limiting factors that prevent that person from achieving optimal health and educate them on the tools they need to help them succeed. Maintaining a healthy weight is dependent on five key factors: food selection, caloric intake, sleep, stress and activity level - all of which are covered by The Health Bible. Once change has begun, the body starts to heal itself, and the need for medication and specialized assistance is no longer necessary. This process has been designed to keep people on track, while complementing their changes in lifestyle. The Health Bible places basic nutritional strategies at its core, helping people to understand that good nutrition and fitness affect us both mentally and physically.

5
FREQUENTLY ASKED QUESTIONS

That all being said, where do we start? Lets get the creative juices flowing before moving forward into the guts of The Health Bible and how I did it. When public speaking my answers are very open minded and holistic in nature, the same with what you are about to read. Let's start by going through some of the most commonly asked questions my trainers and I get asked daily. If you like what I have to say, the Ten Health commandments will be a great place for you to start. The following is strictly my opinion and should not be taking as gospel.

Why do I have frequent colds and flus?
This is a big one! The first thing I'd say is that you're not sick; you're thirsty! Start drinking more than 3 bottles of water a week and you'll likely get better. Not to mention if you're eating unhealthy, your immune system is not going to be able to fight off the viruses or bacteria that live in you right now. Personally, I believe that the flu season doesn't even exist - it's a giant money-making scheme for Big Pharmaceutical! My thoughts on this are

just thoughts, but I look at it this way: there are 75 trillion cells in the human body and they are outnumbered by other micro-organisms 1-10. That means over 90% of your biomass isn't even you! You're basically a walking ecosystem of both good and bad types of bacteria, all fighting against each other. Crazy, huh? I honestly don't think we really pick up a lot of colds. Rather our bodies don't have the ability to battle what's already inside us due to a weak immune system.

Why is my digestion so brutal?

Think about this, one teaspoon of dirt has over 100,000 micro-organisms in it, and we're identifying more all the time. It's the same with your digestive tract and the different types of bacteria living inside it. A healthy person should have about 2lbs of intestinal flora (other lifeforms) in their digestive tract. Pro and Prebiotics are these bacteria and are tossed on every label in the dairy section. The truth is, there is so much hype about probiotics nowadays, we have forgotten about prebiotics and how they work. Lets keep it simple, the "Pro" and "Pre" concept is like the "Yin" and "Yang." One cannot exist without the other - day cannot exist without night. Your digestive tract is similar to this and is best understood like a garden. A garden is not completely healthy without weeds! A healthy garden needs the weeds to fight off the insects and other things that can harm the plants residing within. When the weeds in the garden die, they provide the nutrients for the plants to grow again and vice versa.

We don't get enough of these micro-organisms in our diet, and that's why its important to reintroduce them..

Nature gave us everything we need, but that marketing departments for grocery stores think you need fruit and veggies to glisten before you'll think of buying them. In the beginning days of my juice bar, we would receive our produce in boxes covered with wax. Someone thought it was a great idea to spray on the fruits and veggies a nice layer of "makeup" to bring out their natural beauty.

How often should I see my doctor?

Trips to the doctor and different specialists usually lead to a cycle that goes on and on. The more need for medication you claim, the more the healthcare system is changing your mind and body chemistry. Don't let your first step be to medicate! Take a look at your nutrition first and consider alternative methods of therapy in conjunction with modern medicine.

Is medication bad for me?

According to the media, there seems to be a need for medication the moment you are feeling depressed, have a headache or simply aren't feeling well. However, there are ways to recover from these symptoms if we are honest about the quality and quantity of exercise and nutrition we receive. Often, when you start to make healthy choices, things seem to improve.

I learned some interesting philosophies while I was living in China. Did you know in some Chinese provinces, traditional doctors will be paid based on how infrequently they see their patients? Meaning the less you have see your doctor, the better he is doing and therefore, the more he is compensated. Whether that compensation is a higher salary or hugs from a panda, well, that's not the point. The point is that, in Western Society, we have our values reversed. Every time you see the doctor, whether it's to get a check-up or a doctor's note, you have to swipe your health card. Booya! They get paid! So where's the incentive for you to stay healthy and medication free?

What is Organic food?

There are many different standards on what constitutes "true organic," but from what I have researched, true organic means that you don't grow anything in the soil for at least three years and you rotate the crop every three months.

Food is really only as good as the soil you grow it in. Nitrogen, phospherous and potassium are the three big macronutrients that plants get from the soil. If you grow something in the same soil repeatedly, eventually you deplete the nutrients from the soil. At this point, there's nothing good left in it for plants to grow. This leaves only one option, fertilizer. We reintroduce these macronutrients in the form of fertilizer in order to grow anything in the soil. Since these macronutrients are artificially introduced, plants in this soil are going to grow rapidly. That being said, the plant will not have a strong immune system. Herbicides, fungicides, and pesticides are then used to fight off the things which the plant would normally be able to cope with. By this point, we have multiple synthetic chemicals that are harmful for us and the plant, just so we can get the food to hit shelves fast enough to make that bottom line.

This decrease in food quality can be directly linked to the increase in population, which forced the development of quicker, easier ways to grow, store, and sell food.

The way food is packaged can be expensive to companies as well., Health Canada charges $25,000 per product to have an "All-Natural" label placed on the product, while the organic label itself at times can cost an astounding $55,000.

What's wrong with Soy and GMO foods?

I don't know everything about Genetically Modified Organisms (GMO), but I can say that after working with hundreds of clients, there's a good chance they are a long-term problem. Remember, this is from my perception as a nutritionist. Multinational food and agriculture companies invest in producing genetically modified foods to create a product that doesn't require a ton of pesticides, will grow faster, produce more bountiful harvests, and above all else, gives them the potential of obtaining a patent.

Soy products are a great example of an understandable GMO product. The soy plant typically requires a lot of water to grow, but if there are any weeds nearby, the soy plant doesn't get enough water. The plant can be altered genetically to make growing ideal. From what I have read about the genetically modified preparation of soy, an overabundance of isoflavone is created throughout the process. Isofavone in large doses can affect your hormone levels and is where soy gets its "bad reputation." Naturally grown soy, however, is a great source of protein. To conclude, the old saying still rings true: "Buy fresh, buy local."

Should I follow the food guide?

If you take a nutrition course in Canada these days, you're likely going to follow a food guide which was put together by our government. To create the Canadian food guide, they hired Kraft Canada, who have modified the guide only twice (despite medical breakthroughs) since it was first launched some time ago. If you're Kraft Canada and you're going to tell 34 million people how to eat, what are you going to do? Create a good business model, and base it around products your company produces! Sure they advertise the nutrient content of their foods, but is it as simple as following a nutrient-centered-diet?

What you have to understand about nutrients is that it's more about portion control and nutrient timing than anything else. Unfortunately the food guide has too many starchy carbohydrates. If it were up to me, I would take the total servings of starchy carbs and replace them with more wholesome, worthwhile fruit and veggie carbs instead. Juicing is an important part of the process because it simplifies the consumption you need to achieve optimal health. Without it, you'll be eating approximately 14 fruits & veggies a day and for most of us, that's no easy task.

Should I care about my weight?

Weighing yourself tells you nothing about your actual health. When you get emotionally attached to your weight, you end up with negative thoughts and added stress. Good nutrition is all about hormones and cortisol (the stress hormone) control. When you get up in the morning and you jump on the scale and get upset about it, you've just ruined your day. The negative effect of that one brainwave creates a cortisol and white blood cell release. It takes your body at least 27 hours to filter cortisol through the kidneys and liver which, in the end, creates more body fat. Your mindset has everything to do with it! It's not just about counting calories and pounds on a daily bases.

Let's break down your overall weight into four categories, lean muscle, body water, body fat and bones and connective tissues. We all know muscle weighs more than fat, so if weight loss alone is important to you, stop eating and drop the heaviest stuff you can, your muscle. Weight loss should never be done this way. I've worked with people who think they have lost an amazing amount of weight.. However, when I take their body composition, their lean muscle mass and resting heart rate is so low I do a double take to make sure they are not a zombie. By this point, we are probably looking at permanent damage to the body. Focus on reducing your body fat mass alone, while keeping your body water nice and high.

6
TAKE A BRAIN DUMP

Often, our biggest problem is ourselves and our self-sabotage. My brother once told me, "If you really want to know what your problem is, just look in the mirror!" The following questions will help you create and maintain a positive connection to your lifestyle change. Take some time and answer them honestly, it's only going to help you in the long-run.

- What activities must you do every year?
- What activities must you do every 6 months?
- What activities must you do every month?
- What activities must you do every week?
- What activities must you do every day?
- What does your perfect day look like?
- What would you accomplish in that day?
- How many hours would you work?
- How much uninterrupted time would you have?
- How much time would you spend on technology?
- What other aspects would make it a perfect day?
- What's the most important thing for you to do?
- What are the most important roles you play?

- What is your most productive time?
- What would be your most creative time?
- What are you willing to have other help you with?
- What are you really living for?
- What do you hope to accomplish?

This particular exercise has made my life easier and can do the same for you. Write out three or four lines for each question and feel free to write off the page. Now, write it a second time and make sure that every goal you write down is unreasonable. The goal is to get you out of your normal thought-process which is usually very self-limiting.

I want you to get this now and also save you some headaches. You do have to write things out in order to achieve them. It's just like studying, and the universe rewards effort! It doesn't matter if you are counting beans in a factory, or taking the extra time to shovel snow off the corners of the drive way. It's said that everything is "made in China". Have you actually ever thought of the amount of people, and how much time and effort is involved in producing something as simple as an oven or a pencil? The amount of energy is incalculable, but these daily items are amazing and change our everyday life. Next time you vacuum, instead of sucking up the pennies, pick them up and you'll start attracting wealth. Try it! It doesn't matter what you do. Simply karma at work!

When you start tediously writing down your goals and keeping track of what you're eating, you'll start holding yourself accountable to not eating Pop-Tarts, Kraft Dinner, or KFC. As we get older, it's not that things start to slow down, it's more that we settle into our bad habits more and more. We become more settled into who we are on a deeper level and it becomes more difficult to change. We get lazy, comfortable and less grateful for the simple things. My uncle once told me, "The older we get, the more we become who we truly are." That's scary! Eventually, it all starts to catch up with us. Most people that I meet under 25 don't care much about what they eat or put into their bodies. Eventually, they'll care once they start to notice things change, and not for the better. Now look, I don't want to come into this by scaring you, but I've found that a little bit of fear can help motivate people to change for the better.

You probably don't need a complete diet overhaul, but maybe with a little renovation you'll start to see that the little things do count! Whether it's cutting-out a soda or adding an apple, you'll notice that the little things really do make a big difference.

This book should be seen as an open discussion with yourself. I'm really here to answer your questions and you can send me an email at any time. "The most stupid question is the one that is not asked." I know this sounds cliché, but it's true.

Take a look at some of these common symptoms of poor nutrition and highlight any with which you identify.

- Slow metabolism
- Low energy
- Fatigue
- Energy highs and lows

- Poor sleep
- Skin problems
- Sugar cravings
- Frequent colds, flu, etc.
- Frequent trips to the doctor/specialist
- Need for medication
- Suggested behavioral problems

There's a common theme here: All of these symptoms are heavily elevated by overconsumption of sugar and starchy carbohydrates.

Pick one of the 10 Commandments in the next section and make a commitment to stick with it for at least 21 days before changing anything else. At that point, your body will start to adapt physiologically and, hopefully reduce some of these symptoms. Most times when I am coaching someone on a one-on-one basis, I suggest starting on the first one, and only moving forward to the next step when you have fully mastered the one you are on.

It's a really good idea to make an appointment for a checkup with your doctor. Let him or her know you are thinking about making some changes to your diet and would like to be sure it's a good idea with your present situation. They will likely do some blood work to check for normal balances of PH, vitamins and minerals. All things I think can give us some feedback on general health.

Your Brain Dump exercises, a trip to your doctor, and the Ten Health Commandments are the best starting point you can give yourself. Next, I will be explain the formula I use to initiate change in a prioritized order. It doesn't matter if you're an average Joe or an Olympic athlete. The basics are the basics, and there is always room for improvement.

7

THE TEN HEALTH COMMANDMENTS

Over the years, I've tried to figure out my own psychology, and why is seems that we all have the similar problems. I had a moment of clarity while speaking with clients that changed everything. I perfectly summed up our common exercise problem with a simple thought, "The longer we go from our last workout, the harder it is to get the next one done."

From that point, I focused on finding strategies to help us through some common issues. What I'm about to share with you are the strategies that worked for myself and hundreds of others. Over the years, I've managed to pull together a team of doctors, pharmacists, nutritionists, juice bartenders, life coaches, and top experts on behavior modification. I've tried to find solutions for every problem I've come across. The following is a list of strategies that will help you get leverage for change. Leverage is taking something small and using it to move something big. With these simple health strategies, it is recommended you start at the beginning, and only move forward once you have completely mastered that step.

Live One Meal At A Time - Eat Every 2-3 Hours

This is a big one, and seems much easier than it actually is because of the amount of time it takes to do groceries and cook everything up. There are a lot of hidden time consumer's with this step, such as, packing lunches and snacks, and cleaning all the containers only to re-pack them again the next day.

No matter what the goal, the get started advice stays the same. Don't worry so much about what you're eating as much as when you're eating. Don't make any drastic changes to your diet just yet. Start recording everything you eat in a food journal and focus on eating more frequently. Eat like you did before, but just start eating every 2-3 hours and log it all in your food journal. If you want to eat donuts and brownies, do it! However, be sure to record it in your journal! Of course I'm giving you an extreme scenario here, but if you calculate how many hours there are in your day, you'll see there is a lot of meals and snacks to get in. You'll see moving through the Ten Health Commandments that once you start eating more frequent meals, we can start to focus on making the right choices.

For starters I can say for overall health and an ass-kicking physique, you'll need strategies designed specifically around eating every 2-3 hours. I can tell you from my experience, 80% of your results will come from this step alone, and that's why I'm telling you about it first. The quickest & easiest way to increase your meals is to start making healthy smoothies & juices. Having two a day, on top of your standard 3 meals will boost your metabolism so high your body will flush out the extra body fat as a result, not to mention you're getting higher water content in your food, and it takes less time.

Your body chemistry is still living in the Stone Age. That means that we are supposed to eat as we were a long time ago. Early man would essentially eat whatever we could find, and spend all day looking for food. Berries, nuts, seeds and uncooked meat may not sound appetizing, but it's the delivery of food to the body in this way that is fascinating to me.

I'm all about time with my approach because we are living in such a fast paced world that I don't think most are ready to face the reality here. Someone's job and family responsibilities go to the core of who they are. That's why I have everyone start with the Brain Dump exercise. If you haven't completed it yet, turn the T.V. off and get it done. If I can go from nothing to where I am now, mainly because of the Brain Dump exercise, it will also work for you. If it was appropriate to, I'd swear here to get you to take action.

First Things First - Get Alkaline

Like a modern day caveman, start carrying some apples, bananas, and small bags of carrots with you through the day. Easy right? Start including a serving of fruit or vegetables with every meal. This gives you consistent energy, helps you get alkaline, helps you detox every meal and drop body fat. But wait! I think I've hear of this alkaline thing before. Remember when I mentioned last chapter to get your blood work done to check for the balance of vitamins, minerals and P.H.? Think back to chemistry class. If you can remember there is a scale that is used to measure substances for acidic or alkaline properties.

The human body has different areas of different P.H. balances, but the blood is the most important! Our blood has an optimal P.H. level that it should be at for all of the body's functions and processes to be normal. Think of when you open a pool up after the winter. You check the water, which is usually pretty acidic from all the crap sitting in it through the season. In order to rebalance the water to the right P.H. for a dip, you go to the pool store, and they give you a bucket of Calcium to toss in. Calcium neutralizes water, bringing it from an acidic P.H. to a more neutral alkaline state. The body works in a similar way. When your blood is acidic, the body will do anything it can to neutralize itself back to the right P.H. balance. The body slowly robs calcium from the bones, and magnesium from your tissues to keep your blood at the sweet spot, nut short of neutral in the alkaline zone. In fact there is a lot of scientific information I could give you on other ways to check your P.H. balance but I want to keep it simple and move on to the more important facts like, what changes the P.H. of your body.

If you are what you eat, then the foods we eat are the main reason we are either acidic or alkaline. For the most part, fruits and vegetables are Alkaline forming in the system, where meat and chemically processed foods are acidic forming. What is extremely important to remember is the verdict is not yet out on how to determine if a food is acidic or alkaline. Scientists have used a few different methods to measure whether or not foods substances are of either side. Some tests will take a piece of food matter, burn it to an ash, then test it in distilled water. Others say that method in itself changes the chemistry too much to accurately designate a specific P.H.

Common sense would suggest lemons and grapefruits are acidic, and they are sitting in your fruit bowl. However these particular examples are generally alkaline forming to the system. Everything breaks down and changes once it enters the body. The small intestine is the most acidic place in the human body. Everything has to pass through here, so you would think anything that passes through becomes acidic but the body chemistry is much more complex then we need to know at this point.

Now I know what you are thinking... Why are we focusing so much on fruits & vegetables (carbohydrates) instead of proteins and fats proteins? The answer is simple! Fruits and veggies are alkaline forming to the system, and when the body is alkaline it detoxes properly and makes it difficult for disease to set in. The majority of people I meet simply do not get enough alkaline fruits and vegetables, thus their body is not at homeostasis, or in harmony. Strive for 60% of your diet to come from alkaline foods. Be sure you're alkalizing your body every 2-3 hours so you can reduce your risk of disease and allow your body to detox itself properly every meal, day by day.

When eating out, I only order from the entrees which have an option of substituting fries or potatoes for veggies. As mentioned in step one, if you want to eat brownies, that's fine! Just have a serving of veggies or fruit with them! The best way to eat more fruits and vegetables is to pick up a juicer or blender. Start making juices and smoothies every day to keep it interesting and save on time. The first time I started doing this, my body reduced its inflammation drastically and began to show amazing fat loss results right away. This gave me a dose of motivation, and some momentum moving forward.

I did find another healthy solution that worked so well, I decided to get into the juice bar business. I discovered juice cleansing as a form of detoxing and getting alkaline. You have the option to either start incorporating fruits & veggies into every meal, or start doing a juice cleanse detox and continue juicing when you're done. Regardless of what you do, it's best to first clean the crap food out of your kitchen and replace it with ingredients you can use to make healthy smoothies and juices. When you set up a No-Fail Environment, you're less likely to eat the stuff you shouldn't. Doing a juice cleanse detox has always been my #1 recommendation for anyone starting a new program because it worked so well for me. During that time, you'll start to curb your cravings for sugars and starches and definitely give yourself a foundation upon which you can build. Before you move forward with your juice cleanse, I suggest running it by your doctor. It's essentially a "lower-protein" diet because there is no meat or dairy consumed during the process. After your cleanse, you can begin to boost your protein levels to optimal levels.

Practice, Not Perfection - Have Protein Every Meal

Plain and simple: people just don't get enough protein after an overall examination of their food journal! If you're anything like me, it took me years to develop the self-discipline to cook and eat a chicken breast with every meal. Spices are your best friend, and you should be using them to spice up your food and keep things interesting. There are lots of other ways you can get protein into your diet, and it's learning these little meal tricks that can help you come out on top in the end. Once you learn what protein is and where else you can find it, these little first base hits defiantly add up. Getting enough protein into your diet really boils down to cooking and managing your time to do so. I spend at least a few hours a week pre-cooking all my meat for the week ahead. That way its super easy for me to toss a chicken breast or two into a lunch salad. I suggest following the grocery list I provided and pick up a variety of different protein sources like turkey, beef, eggs and fish.

Without getting to deep into the biochemistry of the body, protein is made of what we call amino acids. There are a total 20 amino acids, some are essential for the body, others not so much. The term "a complete protein" means it has all of the amino acids that are needed for the body to break it down and deliver it to your muscles. Meats and animal products usually have these complete proteins, and while some fruits, vegetables, nuts and seeds also have amino acids, they are usually missing a few. It is this reason vegetarians should be knowledgeable in this area, so they can combine the right foods to get all 20 amino acids.

When you're not getting all the amino acids that your body needs, it will go into protein deficiency (after about three months) and you will lose your energy, sex drive and hormonal balance. You will also likely start to lose your lean muscle mass, simply because you're not getting enough amino acids to support the muscle you already have. This doesn't mean you need to go out and break the bank on protein supplements. I have met a lot of people who automatically associate the word protein with fitness and a slim trim body. Maybe so, but remember I did put fruits and vegetables before this step. Supplements can give you an awesome edge, especially when you start exercising, and I recommend picking some up to begin with so you can boost your protein levels. By simply making two shakes a day to consume on your break, you are consuming more vitamins, minerals, and of course the most important factor, water!

Everyone needs protein and you need something that is fast, easy and tastes great. This is why we have a 2.6 billion dollar supplement industry on our hands, a nutrition house on every corner, and empty promises on the T.V. commercials that promote them. You need to get a protein supplement that tastes amazing when you're choosing one, not just okay. Ask for some samples and most stores will let you return it if you really don't like it. You can't be a push over if you're going to try this. Take the time to talk with the protein pusher about what products have the best flavor technology. If you get something you have to convince yourself you like because of your newest health crazy, you won't use it long. Settle with something that tastes amazing, even with water, and something that mixes well. How many people do you know have a bucket of protein underneath the sink or on top of the fridge with dust on the lid? Everyone! The industry has come a long since the early 2000s, and most supplements taste and mix better than they ever did before.

After some research, I began to notice that some of the ingredients in these products were harmful to the body. There is an entire section later on in The Health Bible that outlines this in detail, and will blow your mind. At this stage, however, my motto is it's better to get something rather than nothing, and reduce the harm of protein deficiency. You can eventually start to remove these products and begin getting protein from natural sources, but not until you have first taken the time to truly master this habit. As you get into this habit, don't always believe that more protein and scoops are better. Start simple by having a few smoothies each day or by adding a scoop here and there in your oatmeal to get your intake higher than it was. Depending on your body's ability to assimilate this protein, you will likely only be able to digest around 21 grams per sitting.

Sweat Everyday - Carbs Are Exercise Earned

Most people exercise in a way that creates a lot of pain in their body both physically, and psychologically. That's why most people don't keep consistent with their workouts. If you follow the old principle of "No Pain No Gain," all you're doing is building an association of pain to something that is absolutely ideal for your body. This is not a philosophy I recommend, so don't get too hung up with workouts or exercises you think you should be doing on that video you got last Christmas. Simply focus on finding ways to sweat at least once a day. If you really want to lose fat, you'll have to earn those starchy carb meals by sweating first! Sweating everyday boosts your metabolism and helps your body assimilate nutrients, and eliminate wastes. As you read on you may be a little surprised to learn something as simple as breathing can elevate both of these processes tremendously. When you sweat, your body begins to move what is called the lymphatic system. This system has no pump and is considered to be the sewage and waste highway of the body in that it is responsible for flushing out toxins through your sweat glands. Think of it as the pipes that run under the streets of a city. When we don't sweat on a regular basis the pipes get clogged up and need to be flushed out.

Physical activity can be broken down into two categories, anaerobic and aerobic. Resistance training is considered to be anaerobic activity, which means we are using the muscles of the body to resist gravity with either our own body weight or dusty equipment we find in our basement. Aerobic activity is Latin, and literally means "with oxygen." These are the types of activity we would consider to be cardiovascular training in which our breathing is elevated and your heart is pumping. Whether its cardio, resistance training, hot yoga, a set of pushups, for now it doesn't matter. Just move the blood around before indulging in your gluten gluttony.

Most people have heard of gluten, but most cannot tell you what they know about why you shouldn't ingest it. From my own perception of the average person's body, I can say gluten brings on inflammation. Yes, there are a lot of other factors like lack of water which could be attributed to the bloating effect, but removing gluten definitely helps drop inches. Everyone's body chemistry is different and some people are allergic to foods that others are not. In regards to gluten this is called Celiac disease. You may not be diagnosed Celiac, however that doesn't mean you won't have a reaction when you ingest gluten.

The allergic reaction can simply be a little inflammation around the waist instead of the neck. Your body's reaction to gluten can vary and is dependent on your body chemistry and genetic makeup. Think of it as only being mildly allergic, not in desperate need of an inter-muscular injection of epinephrine or a toilet.

If you want to eat bread, pasta, rice, or sugary foods, do it. However, be sure to eat them only after you exercise. When you can go for the whole grain varieties and save them until after you exercise. Your body will thank you. This strategy alone was enough to get me amazing results fast. I've been told this process doesn't distinguish between "good", high fiber carbohydrates and "bad," high sugar, empty-calorie carbohydrates. While this was a valid point, the strategy's main purpose was to get your meal and nutrient timing on track. I'm not trying to advise you to start a low-carb diet. Rather, I use this as a great strategy to start with as I began to build an individualized plan. This plan became a "controlled-carb" diet, where most carbs were from veggies and fruits (plus some carbs from smoothies during exercise and some oatmeal post-exercise). Sure, the description above doesn't make for a great one-liner, but boy does this strategy work! When it comes to body composition change, this carbohydrate timing strategy is the single most-effective strategy I have ever used to kick-start fat loss in people with stubborn and hard-to-remove body fat stores. It also minimizes fat gain in people looking to gain muscle.

I have found this technique works regardless of any theoretical objections people toss at me. And it works very, very well. The strategy alone revolutionized some of my clients' bodies and health profiles. This was when I started to learn that I had to match my nutritional plan to my goals. If you want to lose fat, it's quite obvious that you'll have to eat differently than if you want to gain muscle. However, while there are subtle differences between the two eating styles, the principles remain the same.

To sum it all up: if you want to lose fat, eat starchy carbs only when you deserve to. No exercise, no carbs! (Other than carbs from fruits and veggies, of course!) If you want to gain muscle, make sure to time the carbs properly, although you may relax a bit if you have a hard time gaining weight. Just like grammar, there may be exceptions to the rule in certain situations. Don't stress about them right now.

Fat Is Not Evil – Supplement Healthy Oils

This whole idea that fat is bad has changed over the years more times than I'd like to write about. There is no such thing as a truly evil food, it's the combo of amounts and times that gives it the rap sheet of a criminal. We're taught that fat is a bad thing, but did you know that you actually have to ingest fat to burn fat? If not, the body fat you have becomes extremely stubborn, thus your body will hold on to all it has for dear life. For the average person, roughly 30% of their calories should come from healthy fats. In some cases, this can actually range from 20-40% depending on your individual's body type, as reviewed in detail later on. Remember there are only three macronutrients. So, when you eat low fat, you are eating high protein and carbs. I discuss these situations frequently when working with people one-on-one and it's a common question on our social media. Notice I have covered all three of these within the first 5 Health Commandments.

When looking at fat all in itself there are three types, monounsaturated, polyunsaturated, and saturated fats. The problem is the majority of foods have too much saturated fats. This unbalances the better ones we need to allow everything to metabolize and get used up for energy. One gram of fat has 9 calories or unit of energy per gram. That's more than double from a gram of proteins or carbs. Your body stores fat for precisely this reason, it's a great source of energy! I might be moving into left field here but, the more body fat you have on you, the longer you can survive through a famine that Mother Nature puts us through. Simply the chunkier you are, the more she will love you in the game of survival. I may be getting a little symbolic on you here but fat can't be bad! Especially if the most loving figures we know like Buddha and Santa are the spitting image of that we think we don't want to look like. The following is a list of sources from which we can get our fats from.

Monounsaturated: Avocados, Olive Oil, Nuts and Nut Butters.

Polyunsaturated: Vegetables, Flax Seed Oil, Fish Oils, Nuts and Nut Butters.

Saturated: Meat, Dairy, Eggs, Butter, Cheese, and Coconut Oil.

Remember, in general the type of fats you're eating is much more important than the amount you consume, depending on your self-control. These three different types of fat should be balanced for optimal health. Your fat intake should be 1/3 monounsaturated, 1/3 polyunsaturated, and 1/3 saturated fats. Yes, we're taught to fear saturated fats but, when saturated fat intake is balanced with a healthy amount of monounsaturated and polyunsaturated fats, you don't have to be afraid of it. Eating this way is easier than it looks, especially if you start supplanting. In regards to your diet, focus on adding the healthier nuts, seeds, and fish oil supplements into your diet of fruits and veggies and everything should balance itself right out. Once I started looking into fish oils, I learned that having a few capsules of these beauties with every meal would re-balance everything out, help reduce inflammation, and increase brain function. The brain is composed of mainly fatty tissue so that should speak volumes about the importance of fat in your diet.

I recommend that everyone include fish oil supplements in their nutrition plan. Fish oil, flax, or hemp seed oil (for vegetarians) help improve your body composition. Supplementing these oils help you lose fat, look leaner, and protect against heart disease, cancer, and diabetes. So take your fish oil; go for a solid 6 grams or 6 capsules a day. Leave them on your desk or put them in your washroom so you don't forget to take them. Flax & hemp seed oil both require refrigeration in a dark bottle to prevent them from oxidizing and going rancid from light and temperature exposure. Pick up a small bottle from a health food store, odds are you'll use it before it can go bad. When shopping at the bulk food store, be mindful of how long they have been sitting there for. It's not likely they will be tossing expensive pecans away if they still have uninformed people buying them. Simply put, the higher the oil content of these nuts and seeds will dictate how quickly they go bad. Choices like pecans and walnuts have a higher oil content then something like almonds, which usually have a longer shelf life.

When cooking it's good to me mindful of the amounts of oils you add and the types you use. When in the grocery store you will notice there is a large variety of oils to choose from. Always use unrefined oils and understand that these oils change depending on the temperatures your cooking with. Depending on the type of oil you use, higher temperatures will de-stabilize and oxidize some oils faster than others.

High Heat Frying: 375F/190C
- Palm Oil
- Coconut oil
- Clarified Butter, Ghee
- Lard

Medium Heat Sautéing: 325 F/163C
- Olive Oil
- Sesame Seed Oil
- Hazelnut Oil
- Pistachio Oil

Low Heat: 212 F/100C
- Sunflower Oil
- Safflower Oil
- Pumpkin Oil

Little To No Heat: Up To 120F/49C
- Hemp Oil
- Flax Oil
- Cod Liver Oil
- Borage Oil

If you wear the pants in the family and thus do most of the cooking, refer back to this list before you purchase a 10 liter jug of canola oil from Costco. You don't want to lose all the benefits of healthy oils just because you like to scorch everything in the oven. When frying, always put your oil into a cold pan, then turn the heat up gradually.

Keep It Simple - Carry A Water Bottle Everywhere

An average of 65% of the body is water, the brain is composed of about 70% water, and the lungs are nearly 90 percent water. You don't just need water to run your body optimally, you need it to survive! Lack of water can lead to dehydration, a condition that occurs when there isn't enough water in the body to carry on with normal functioning. I know its rocket science eh? Here is the kicker though, even mild dehydration can destroy your energy levels and leave you feel exhausted and dyeing for a coffee or cupcake pick me up. So how much water do you need, not just to kick away dehydration, but to maintain your health and consistent fat loss efforts? Consume roughly one-half your weight in ounces of pure water each day. For example, if you weigh 160lbs, you should consume 80oz of fresh water daily for optimal health.

Some factors that increase your need for additional water are exercise, hot environments like California living, or certain health conditions. Simply feeling thirsty isn't a reliable gauge of your body's need for water. The first thing I look for to quickly gauge someone's level of dehydration is dry lips. A better check on hydration, as wild and unpleasant as it may sound, is the color of your urine. Clear or light-colored urine means you're well hydrated, and dark yellow or amber color usually signals dehydration. Of course there are all the milder signs of dehydration that you may never have considered such as tiredness, dry mouth, muscle weakness, muscle spasms, headache, dizziness, or lightheadedness. The list can go on and on simply because water is everything to the body and its overall energy.

The solution really is that simple, carry a bottle around with you everywhere! This seems to be the newest fashion statement. I suggest you make it the same for you. But before I get into how to choose one, I do have to say that I do retain approximately 7 bottles a month at Optymal Health Studios because of people forgetting them around the juice bar. That's eighty four bottles a year, and some of them could be yours. The point I'm trying to drive across here is you will misplace your bottle if that's all it is to you. Pick up a bottle that you absolutely love. Go for one made of glass, stainless steel, or something with cartoon characters on it. If you love your bottle you won't leave it behind. I have a few bottles that I love, but my favorite is a green, one liter Gatorade bottle with a squirt top. I prefer the squirt top bottles because I have found through measuring my intake, I consume much more water with this style of lid.

If you work in an office where you have access to a water cooler, great! Bring your bottle with you and continue to fill it up as much as possible. Your co-workers may wonder why you're making additional trips to the washroom, but your body will eventually get used to your newer level of hydrating, and the urge to pee every time you drink will slow. It's all about optimizing your health and they will soon see a BIG differences in your body and your energy. Make a goal to drink 5-6 (8 oz.) bottles or cups of water during your workday, and then 2-3 in the evening. Have fun with it! Get an app on your phone that measures how much water you get or just set your alarm every few hours as a reminder to fill it up. Just make sure you get a water bottle you love, you're less likely to forget it at the gym or office. Be patient because I took me a few years to really get consistent with reminding myself day in and day out.

Now for your next goal: eliminate garbage concentrated juices & sodas from the store. If it doesn't go through a juicer or blender in your kitchen, the living enzyme components are totally dead, and so is that beverage to you. The same goes for coffees and teas full of cream and sugar. Focus on only drinking fluids that are zero calories! While many people believe that fruit juice is a healthy alternative to soda, unnatural fruit juices have little nutritional value. Of course, there is one time when these juices can be useful. That's right: during and after exercise when you need to replenish your body. Beyond these, stick with H2O not just from the tap, but from your high water content foods as well. In the end, the best water you can consume is the water that is contained in these living foods. This is your new golden standard in terms of water. It's been filtered by the plant, filled with all the nutrients that your body needs, and is much better than tap water polluted with chemicals.

This leads me into my next point about water. There are lots of studies and conspiracy theorist talking shop about this. As mentioned before, most that have something to say, are likely dehydrated themselves. Without getting to deep into the details myself I can say you should try and stay away from highly chlorinated water as much as possible. Since your body is roughly 65% water, you want the water you drink to be as pure as possible for physiological functions, disease prevention, performance, and ideal body composition. On average, you should drink 8-12 cups per day and at least 14 cups a day for fat loss. That's 3.6 liters a day! Although the water consumed in your juices, recovery drinks, or green tea counts, relying on these drinks alone is not the way to go. You may have to "top off" with some clean, high-quality H2O. All in all the best way to get yourself closer to your 3.6 litter goal is to practice this ninja trick every day, and I will share it with you now as I do with all the people I work with. Every morning when you wake up, as soon as your feet touch the floor go straight to the kitchen and drink a bottle or two of water. That is upon raising and that means you will literally still be half asleep by the time the bottle touches your lips. You should be clearing the sleep from your eyes and going for the shower only after you put it back. As your body sleeps it goes through the physical and mental recovery processes and the byproducts of this is a lot of waste that need to be eliminated in the morning. Most of this waste can collect itself in the stomach, that's why starting your day with a healthy amount of water can be so helpful not just for hydration, but for recovery.

Plan Ahead - Prep Your Food The Night Before

The hardest part about eating well isn't understanding which foods are good and which are bad. It's making time to prepare your meals and staying consistent! If you fail to plan, you plan to fail and nothing could be farther from the truth. Sometimes, good nutrition is less about the food and more about making sure the food is available when it's time to eat every 2-3 hours.

You're going to need to come up with food preparation strategies in order to ensure that you can consistently get what you need, when you need it. Now that you have a good handle on living one meal at a time, and combining your carbs, fats and proteins, you should dive into the recipe section and start planning ahead. Whether that means cooking a bunch of chicken on Sunday for the upcoming week, or prepackaging salads into Tupperware containers, it all helps. All of this is a big step in the right direction especially if you have had your mother in law feeding you pork sausage every night before bed. Take this time to put yourself first and pack those meals, and pack them good! Similarly, in the morning, get up thirty minutes earlier, drink a liter of water and have a smoothie or high protein breakfast. Most people give me the excuse that they don't have time in the morning. The answer is simple, get up 10-30 min earlier and don't go to bed with the T.V. on until one A.M. I've gone as far as to time myself making my staple six meals and looking for shortcuts to keep prepping time to a minimum. Let me give you an example of how fast some meals can be in reality.

Cooking steel cut oats should be done the night before because they take some time to soften up for you eat them. Cook them in a crock pot or on the stove the night before so it's ready to go in the morning. If you're not a fan of steel cut oats, go for the large plain oats. Turn the tap water onto hot and let it run while you get the pot out and put it onto the stove top on high. By the time you get back to the running water it's already halfway to boiling, measure out one cup of water, dump it in the pot, and get your oats. Oatmeal is awesome because it's one cup of water, to one cup of oats. By the time you measure out your oats, the water will be boiling, toss in some frozen berries, protein powder, and cinnamon, then mix it up! Take it off the heat and cover wail you go fix your hair up for the day. It will take you less time to cook oatmeal then it did for me to type this up here. If eggs are more your style that's great, they take just as much time or less following the same method providing you chopped up your greens the night before. As the old cliché very accurately states, "failing to plan is planning to fail."

When you eat out, you have little to no control over which chemicals and oils are added to the food to make it taste better. Not to mention you have no control of the quality of the ingredients they use, especially when it comes to fruits and vegetables. To keep it simple, better quality foods mean more vitamins and minerals. No vitamin pills can even come close to matching the vitamins, minerals, and living enzymes that good ol' fruits and veggies contain. Aim to eat a real meal with lean meats, veggies, high fibers, and good fats. Of course, you won't have whole food meals prepared for every day, but if there's one thing I've learned, you get back what you put into things. Sure, it's much easier to grab an energy bar, a handful of mixed nuts, granola bar, or a protein shake than it is to prepare a whole meal. However, it's best to get as many whole food meals in your diet as possible. Eat bars and drink shakes only when you're crunched for time or during your post-exercise period for liquid nutrition.

Early To Bed, Early To Rise – Have A Big Breakfast

Very few average people understand the connection between their body shape and what they slam down their pie hole on autopilot every meal. It's easier to think of most people body shape as pretty much a large triangle with the tip at your head, and the base wide at the hips. Symbolically, they eat the same way with a very small breakfast of express and a muffin, followed by a good lunch, and a massive dinner. Starting to see the connection here? Let's reverse the psychology here and flip that baby around making our breakfast the largest meal, getting smaller through the day, and giving you that V cut around the midsection. There has been a lot of debate about this one out there. I have heard from some of the best in my field, and seen what works for others. Not to mention, there are a lot of complex nutritional digestive research in this area sending conflicting messages, and confusing everyone into analysis paralysis. My rule of thumb is to have your biggest meals earlier in the day (high to low glycemic) so they are in rhythm with your hormonal levels and body clock. Simply enough, if you're not a big eater in the morning, eat something until you're full and then come back to it as a snack later.

Good nutrition is all about hormone and cortisol control as is later discussed in The Health Bible. Cortisol is known as the stress or junk food hormone. However this hormone fluctuates up and down through our twenty four hour clock to wake us up in the morning and put us to bed when it's at a lower level in the evening. Cortisol levels are highest in the morning between six and 9 A.M. which means your metabolism is stimulated and your body is hungry for nutrients after fasting through the night. While on the topic of fasting, and in an extreme opposite example, even not eating food (fasting) can be healthy and detoxifying in some instances. Not to mention, getting hungry every now and then can actually help you get over being a picky eater. Children that act fussy about food have usually not experienced that many hunger pains.

If you have your biggest meal in the morning, make it good, and high in protein, it will help keep your stress hormones and cortisol levels lower through the day and up until bed time when everything starts to get ready for rest and recovery. Eat like a king for breakfast, a queen for lunch, and a prince for dinner. In other words, eat your largest meal in the beginning of the day and your smallest meal before bed. All of these hormones wind down through the day up until 10 P.M. when our natural sleep hormones increase. Your digestion should wind down as well but you should still eat every 2-3 hours, if its bed time and you haven't eaten in 3 hours, eat! But, make it high in protein and low in simple sugars to fuel your recovery through the night.

Go Natural – Shop At The Farmers' Market

By the time you get around to implementing this commandment, you may be knee deep in protein powder and Cliff Bar wrappers. Yes it may get you by the first few commandments and in my opinion, until you really get a master of your cooking and food prep times, use supplements as an edge. The point I want to get across here is to start removing a lot of these supplements because, although the label says it's good, it is still processed heavily. Don't get too addicted to these time savers, you should find yourself at a point where your supplementation is just habit. By this point, bite the bullet and start removing them. I've looked over tons of food journals in my day, and one thing stands out: most of us eat in a very habitual manner. The meals are basically the same things in different ways, over and over again. Breakfasts, lunches, and dinners all use the same "world class" ingredients that led you to get this book in the first place. If you already started your food journal, the similarities will jump out at you.

It's extremely important to start including a variety of seasonal foods into your eating patterns. For most people, the problem is usually not enough fresh vegetables or quality meat. Find a local farmers' market that operates during a time that works with your schedule and get your butt down there every two weeks to change it up. Better yet, find a good butcher that can provide you with a variety of protein sources like venison, bison, wild boar – or maybe some ostrich that was massaged with only the finest oils – instead of the old classics like chicken, beef, and eggs. Don't just opt for the usual fruit and vegetables! Get exotic and incorporate pineapple, mango, berries, apricots, spinach, kale, and cauliflower. Make those salads pop! By doing this, you'll surely be getting higher nutrient-content meals and you'll also foster some nutritional awareness, which is always a good thing. In nature, we weren't provided with convenience food as we are today. If you rotate your foods, you keep your body guessing and your pots and pans will thank you for the new recipe ideas. Use it to help break out of patterns and nutritional ruts from time to time.

When you eat seasonally you are mixing up your food choices according to Mother Earth. It naturally rotates your available choices and mixes things up for your digestive track which can be very helpful for your intestinal flora. Eating in a rotation is beneficial because when foods are in season, they are packed fresh with an abundance of nutrients, usually the ones your body needs that season. Obviously the plants know this!

It's very inexpensive to shop at the farmers market, they appreciate your appreciation, and always welcome your business with smiles and information you can't learn at your average supermarket. Looking towards the future, most farmers markets will be moving into big box grocery stores over the next five years. That seems to be the news business model being written about, not just because of foot traffic, but a new trendy passion for food, and long Canadian winters.

This method of farmers market shopping is a great way to lose weight and should be done once a week. The foods are different all the time and they never have them on the stand for more than one day. In general you can rotate your own choices by only eating particular foods every four days. That means if you eat chicken, you don't eat it until you have completed the rotations full cycle. If you have a hard time committing to this, take it for a test drive first. Write down everything you eat so you can identify your patterns and common foods, then list them out, and start to organize them into your own four day rotation.

Live And Let Live - Plan Your Cheat Meals

Most people are all or nothing with their diet and exercise program. There is no grey area, only on track, or off track. Ditch this idea and get out of the habit of always saying to yourself "I need to get back on track." Most often than not what throws us off are business lunches and social events where others are eating our favorite feel goods. Forget pulling your hair out over this garbage, it's not worth losing sleep over. The winner's mindset should be you, sticking to your plan and not being swayed by others urges to eat crap food. During the week, plan to eat clean and ask others to join you. For the weekends, have your cheat meal and invite them to do the same. At least this way you will not feel the pressure of saying no when invited out to join your coworkers for a heavy cheese stuffed potato. Building up the feeling of neglect in this area can set up binge eating habits and hit or miss diet changes. Eating healthy food and getting pissed off about it gets you nowhere. Your body simply will not be in an ideal state for proper assimilation, let alone enjoyment. If you're used to the feeling of depravation, it can make it hard for you to enjoy a cheat meal. In addition if you eat clean all day every day, it's only a matter of time before you can get bored. The problem is, people are like alcoholics when it comes to cheat days or meals; they can't just have a little bit. The key here is "practice, not perfection." Simply plan ahead and be sure you have a bottle of water handy before going into it so you don't overeat. The fact is unless you are getting ready to stand on the fitness stage in a scandalous bikini, you don't need to be crazy rigid 168 hours a week.

From a psychological perspective, it is important to break the rules every now and again. It's the self-control that you gain coming out of that situation that carries more value anyway. It's like courage, you only get it after the fact. Rather than expecting 100% adherence every day of the week, I suggest 80%. That means that you get to break the rules 20% of the time. Be sure you are clear on what that 20% really means. For example, if you are aiming to consume 1700 to 2000 calories per day, do the math! That's right, you get a 340-400 calorie moment to enjoy. If you decide to eat clean 6 days a week, make your 7th day your cheat day.

A "cheat meal" is a meal that you know isn't on the same path as your overall fitness and health goal. A creamy pasta dinner with a glass of wine is a classic example. Pizza and ice cream for dessert? Yup – that's a cheat meal. If you're anything like me, skipped meals were my biggest problem, and I learned very fast that a skipped meal counts as a cheat meal. If you're trying to drop some body fat, skipping a meal may slow down your progress as your body stores fat. On the other hand, if you're trying to gain muscle, skipping a meal may stunt your results. The same cheat meal may have opposite effects depending on what your goals are. Don't get too hung up with counting cheat meals and worrying about exactly what is or isn't. Just log everything into your food journal and compare it at the end of each week to see how you are doing. If you're not seeing the results you're looking for and your cheat meals are too frequent, you'll know why. Plan your cheat meals and enjoy them. Run with these meals as moments of pleasure, not guilt or shame.

8

THE ULTIMATE BODY TRANSFORMATION SECRET

The single most important thing to do when you start something new is set some goals, and set them high! It's never good to limit or underestimate yourself, especially when it comes to making permanent changes to your body. It's also extremely important to let people know you are embarking on this journey, to help make it official. Make a quick 30 second video of you sharing your current nutritional situation and what you are committing to change; then post it on your social media! Be sure to include your shoe size and marital status so you can be shower in gifts when you achieve your goals! The more uncomfortable you are doing this, the more you should make it happen. Letting go of any subconscious fear of failure is absolutely crucial. Some of the things I ask you to do may sound crazy at times, but if you want to drastically change your situation, I suggest you try them. The rule I follow is this, the more you don't want to tell people you're doing it, the more you should! Get in touch with the 5 people you spend the most amount of time with, outline your health goals, and ask them to support you through it. Better yet, ask them to call you out on it if they see you not following through, especially in public, just to make it a little embarrassing.

It still amazes me how easy and effective this is to write out your goals. In one study, students who were given four weeks to accomplish a goal performed successfully in the following ways:

Students with no written goals – 46%
Students with written goals – 64%
Students who shared goals with friends – 76%

Take special note, that if you don't write or share your goals, you run the risk of average results. I don't know about you, but I look for amazing results, definitely not average! Nobody wants average anymore and I don't blame them. Think about it! Nobody wants average sex, so strive for amazing in everything you do. From what I have seen, people who don't strive for amazing typically fall off the wagon 8-9 times before they become consistent with their meals and workouts.

Before You Start - Establish Your Core Values

The Health Bible core values work for business, relationships and even in the grocery store when you're not sure what to buy. Every time I meet somebody new looking for help, I ask them to write down these core values in their phone or journal. I'm telling you, if you do this, it will make your nutrition and fitness journey so much easier. Apply them to any decision-making process you encounter with your diet and exercise program as we move forward in building this baby.

Live One Meal At A Time – Eat frequently.

First Things First – What is the most important thing to do at that moment?

Practice, Not Perfection – Be accepting that nothing is perfect, and you're doing a good job.

Sweat Once Every Day – Just move the blood, take the stairs, or do a set of push-ups.

Keep An Open Mind – Maybe you don't really know.

Keep It Simple – Overcomplicating things can lead to getting nothing done.
If You Fail To Plan, You Plan to Fail – Plan your meals and workouts each day in the morning.

Think, Think, Think – Don't over think about tomorrow, it never comes.

Easy Does It – Don't change everything all at once.

Live And Let Live – Don't worry about what other people are doing or eating.

Lack Of Accountability

Whenever you work with a trainer they offer you two things: structure and accountability. Structure, in regards to your reps and sets, can be found on the internet or in a magazine. Accountability, however, should come from an external source, at least I the beginning. As time goes on, you being to realize the only person you're really accountable to is yourself. You may have let down your family/friends/trainer/doctor etc. but in the end you're really just selling yourself short.

I came across this article in the early days of my own journey and it literally blew my socks off. Yes, my shoes were on! Here's that article, from Reuters: Study Shows the Value of Food Journaling in Weight Loss; By Will Dunham.

"Keeping a food diary - a detailed account of what you eat and drink and the calories it packs - is a powerful tool in helping people lose weight, U.S. researchers said on Tuesday. The study involving 1,685 middle-aged men and women over a six months period found those who kept such a diary just about every day lost about twice as much weight as those who did not. The findings supported early research that endorsed the value of food diaries in helping people lose weight. Companies including Weight Watchers International Inc. use food diaries in their weight-loss programs. "For those who are working on weight loss, just writing down everything you eat is a pretty powerful technique," Victor Stevens of Kaiser Permanent Centre for Health Research in Portland said in a telephone interview.

"It helps the participants see where the extra calories are coming from, and then develop more specific plans to deal with those situations," said Stevens, who helped lead the study published in the American Journal of Preventive Medicine. The technique also helps hold dieters accountable for what they are eating, Stevens said. The study involved people from four U.S. cities: Portland,

Oregon; Baltimore, Maryland; Durham, North Carolina; and Baton Rouge, Louisiana. Their average weight loss was about 13 pounds (6 kg). But those keeping food diaries six or seven days a week lost about 18 pounds (8 kg) compared to 9 pounds (4 kg) for those not regularly keeping a food diary. "Keeping a food diary doesn't have to be a formal thing. Just the act of scribbling down what you eat on a Post-It note, sending yourself e-mails tallying each meal or sending yourself a text message will suffice," Dr. Keith Bachman, another Kaiser Permanent expert, said in a statement.

Yes, the Ultimate Body Transformation Secret is writing down your goals and everything you put in your mouth! USA Today reported on a similar study, just keeping a simple food diary can double fat loss! That's the reason why every single client at my studio starts with goal-setting and keeping a food journal. If they don't bring it with them, we don't train!

Why This Is So Powerful

Accountability
What's worse than letting down your friends and family? Letting yourself down! When you write your goals, you are forced to answer to yourself at the end of every day. If you commit to writing and tracking your goals each day, you'll quickly get tired of writing about poor results and start doing something about it.

Clarity
As you track your progress, you get a birds-eye view of what you've done and what you need to do to achieve

your health and fitness goals. You are constantly reminding, reviewing and re-planning which gives you a clear path to follow. You're not left guessing and procrastinating.

Motivation

Keeping a daily record is great because anytime you feel down, you can very quickly flip through your journal and see how far you've come; instantly giving you the self-esteem boost you need to keep pushing towards your goals.

Start Your Food Journal

The truth is, most people can't even get a grip on the three BASIC factors that must be in place for any benefits from exercise or eating better to take place. Start here right now and record all of the following as best as you can.

Water Intake – 12-14 cups a day.
Sleep & Wake Cycle – 6-8 hours each night.
Stress Reduction – Yoga, Reiki, Meditation.

Not sure what your food journal would look like? The following takes only minutes a day; holds you accountable and will totally supercharge the choices you make. The first thing you should do each day is get out a pen and write down what you are eating and when you are going to exercise. If you don't write it out, you won't make it real, and it simply won't happen! It only takes a few seconds, and it's exactly how I achieved everything I have done. When you write out what you're eating, you will subconsciously change the decisions you make and how your day goes. Write out exactly what you are going to commit to that day for healthy activity, water, sleep, food and stress reduction.

What To Write In Your Food Journal

Planed Exercise: Hit the gym and take the stairs.
What I Eat: Packed a few things for lunch

8:00AM – Bran flakes and Skim Milk: 250 Calories
9:30AM – Apple: 70 Calories
12:00PM – Chicken Salad & Dressing: 700 Calories
2:45PM – Dirty, Salty Chips: 140 Calories
5:30PM – Big Mac Meal: 1100 Calories
7:00PM – Granola Bar: 120 Calories

Thoughts for Today: Started the day well, but slipped up after the chips I ate at the office. Missed my workout, but walked for 30 minutes after work to make up for it. I'll skip my cheat meal tomorrow and have a healthy meal instead.

Things To Include In Your Food Journal

What You Eat

Don't slack off on the weekends, you want the good, the bad and the ugly. Journaling a few times a week simply isn't good enough because gaps break up the habit-forming process and also give you room to make excuses. For example, you can't miss a day and then say you'll make it up another day. You won't! It's best to write in your journal every day. If you can commit to journaling for 30 days, you'll be hooked! 30 days may seem like a long time, but it'll fly by once you start recording what you do and eat each day.

When You Eat
The easiest thing to do is write what you eat, right after you eat it. The end of the day is a great time to dedicate to filling in the blanks in your journal. It's a good idea to keep your journal by your bed and spend as little as 15 minutes filling it in before putting your head to the pillow or, fill it out while you watch T.V. at night. Whichever you choose, just get 'er done!

Why You Eat It
Writing down why you are eating something specifically can give you some insights into what your body wants you to eat. If you wake up craving peanut butter and toast every morning, asking yourself whether or not it's the peanut butter or the toast can tell you if you need healthy fats (peanut butter) or toast (carbohydrates).

What To Take From This

Again, there's actual proof and testimonials proclaiming how effective keeping a food journal is for transforming your body. If you're serious about getting in great shape and looking better naked, then you absolutely have to try it. It won't become a regret – ever! You have nothing to lose except that spare tire on your waist.

9
DETOX & DIETARY GUIDE

What you need to do with all these meals in your journal is include a serving of fruits or vegetables every time you eat so that you can detox your body and drop additional body fat fast. You're not going to stop craving the foods you're addicted to right away. Therefore, it's a good idea to start carrying some apples or a bag of carrots with you throughout the day so you can banish these guilty pleasures.

If there's something your grandma has been harping on you for years about, it's to eat your damn vegetables! It's about time science has caught up with her. The research has demonstrated that, in addition to the micro-nutrients (vitamins and minerals) packed into veggies, there are also important plant chemicals called "living enzymes" that are essential for optimal physiological functioning. Now, that's a mouthful! Re-read that last sentence so that it can marinate in your head. This is a great way to ensure that you'll never need vitamins: have a serving of fruits and veggies (a serving is 1 cup) with every single snack and meal.

Follow this strategy, and you'll get all the cancer-fighting, free radical-destroying, acid-neutralizing and micro-nutrient-rich power every time you eat.

Vegetables and fruits also provide an alkaline load to the blood. Since both proteins and grains present acid loads to the blood, it is important to balance these acids with alkaline-rich vegetables and fruits. Too much acid and not enough alkalinity means you will have lots of inflammation, a muffin top, loss of bone strength, and muscle mass, which creates the perfect environment for disease to thrive. I could honestly write an entire chapter on being alkaline, but for the purposes of keeping it simple, I recommend that you do your own research. All of the stories you hear about people magically curing themselves of tumors, cancers, and migraines stem from a swift change from acidic to alkaline. So make sure you're alkaline, not acidic!

The best way to do this quickly is to flood the system with juices and smoothies in the form of a juice cleanse. If you're looking for faster results, start one this week for 7 days. Doing a 7-day juice cleanse has always been my #1 recommendation for anyone starting a new program.

Types Of Diets

Regardless of whether or not it's a good time for you to do a detox, we are building you a diet from scratch. It's important for me to explain the pros and cons between all the other diets out there. Humility aside, this way you'll be able to see the wisdom in how this program builds upon itself. Some people think good nutrition means eating fewer sugary desserts and others think it means eating more fruits and vegetables. You may think good nutrition means eating less meat or fewer carbs. All of these are simple to remember, but they are all incomplete.

Low Calorie Diets/Calorie Restriction

Sure, calorie restriction will reduce body weight. Yes, research studies show that extreme calorie restriction in animals can lead to longer life spans. While calorie restriction may lower body weight and perhaps add a few years to your potential life span, it has drawbacks. For starters, long-term restriction can reduce bone density. Did you know that osteoporosis is rampant in young females? These diets can reduce muscle mass and strength, eventually leading to losing independence and mobility with age. Finally, low-calorie diets compromise performance by robbing you of food energy and metabolic power. While a low-calorie diet might help you drop weight, you're mainly losing muscle, not body fat. As you know, muscle weighs more than fat. You'll definitely see declines in your energy levels, health, and performance. The clinical evidence that low calorie diets may help you live longer just isn't well-validated enough in humans, nor are these diets the only way to improve longevity.

Low Carbohydrate Diets

Scientific evidence has shown that these diets could reduce blood sugar and risk of cardiovascular disease, which is generally regarded as "healthy." However, drive those blood sugars too low and you also drive muscle, liver and brain energy too low. If you're active, that's often a recipe for disaster. While very low carbohydrate diets may be healthy in some respects, they will impair most peoples' physical and mental performance. In addition, they can create a very acidic environment within the body – the opposite of what these fruits, veggies and detox ideas will provide for you.

Very High Carbohydrate Diets

High carbohydrate diets that are full of simple sugars, devoid of fiber, and limited in micro-nutrients can improve short term performance in certain sports (especially in endurance sports). In the long run, they can also increase body fat, eventually induce insulin resistance, and even decrease performance.

The Forbidden Fruits And Foods

Depending on whom you live with, you may want to get out a big garbage bag and toss out some of the processed crap you don't need anymore. Anything you can get in a box or from the center aisles in a grocery store is generally designed to have a long shelf life. What that means is they try to remove as much fiber as possible. The higher fiber content foods carry more water on a molecular basis, thus they will go bad quicker than dryer, more processed products. These foods aren't bad, they are just usually eaten in the wrong amounts and at the wrong times.

Please Don't Process That

Forget processed foods packaged in colorful wrappers, boxes, bags, or containers. The quality of a food generally declines in proportion to its degree of processing – especially when "health" claims are made on the label. Your goal is to get as close to original, whole foods as possible. The Optymal Rule: if the food is separated from its original source by more than 3 steps, it's processed! Minimize its contribution to your midsection.

- **Broccoli**: Grows in the ground; 1 step, excellent!
- **Chicken Breast**: Protein from chicken; injected with water; 2 steps, pretty good!
- **Whole Grains**: Grown in the ground; then ground up; 2 steps, cool!
- **Processed Foods**: More than 4 steps! Pretty much anything in the center of the store.

Fatty Meat

Many types of sausage, bacon, and related products are loaded with undesirable types of fat, tons of sodium, and even fillers made of carbohydrates. One of my clients found a prepackaged frozen meatball that offered 15g of protein and 15g of carbs per serving! When I inspected the label, I found that sugar was added to every single meatball! Needless to say, now we stick to turkey meatballs and are wary of processed frozen meats.

Dairy-O

Full-fat dairy products are composed primarily of saturated fat, and can throw off your fatty acid balance and add unnecessary calories. I do make an exception with butter, which is more stable at high cooking temperatures then olive oil (though I'll often use coconut oil, which is also stable at high temperatures).

Frozen Feel-Goods

The low-fat frozen desserts are sugar bombs that drive your insulin levels so high all you want is more within the hour. The obvious ice cream and frozen yogurt products may be low in fat but they are often filled with extra sugars. Be sure to read the label carefully when you're getting your frozen berries too! Just a few months ago, I had to go to the store to get more frozen strawberries for the juice bar. I read the ingredients to find that those babies were laced with 13 grams of sugar! Other juice bar companies and food manufactures sneak sugar in everywhere they can. Sometimes, they will toss these ingredients in oil or sugar water before flash-freezing them to cut back on food costs and make them taste better.

Hard Juice And Soft Drinks

I am asked on a regular basis about orange juice in particular. Just because you get "not from concentrate" doesn't mean it's good for you. Try freshly-squeezed orange juice and compare the taste to the store brand. Huge difference! Although there are many different brands of these beverages, they are owned by a few companies. Orange juice is acquired as a commodity on the Chicago exchange market in frozen bushels. Calorie-containing drinks are one of the biggest contributors to the climbing rates of obesity in this part of the world. It's not just the soda that's the problem. Think that cranberry juice cocktail is healthy? Think again! After water, the second ingredient is sugar. That's why we have NOTHING like that at our juice bar, and I have (unfortunately) turned away customers looking for those types of ingredients. Stick with smoothies, fresh juice, water, green tea, and even a little coffee.

Mayo-Me

Condiments, like mayonnaise, usually contain at least 60% oil and that oil is poor quality (not the healthy fats I recommend). The companies making these foods want to use the cheapest ingredients possible plus many artificial flavorings. Why keep low-value foods in the house at all when you can make your own healthy dressings using olive oil and cider/wine vinegar as a base?

Commercial Un-Dressings

Most bottled sauces are nothing more than spiced high-fructose corn syrup. Toss out the BBQ sauce, ketchup, or spiced vegetable oil. Of course, some sauces can be incorporated into a healthy diet such as salsa, humus, and guacamole. However, you should learn how to spice up your meals naturally without all the extra sugar and calories. Instead of stuffing the fridge with sauces and dressings, stock it with different vinegars and healthy oils like flax and exotic olive oil. Some of my favorite dressings are pesto, liquid amino acids (tastes like soy sauce), salsa, curry sauce, tomato sauce, balsamic vinegar, red and white cooking wine, raspberry vinegar, and spiced flax oil. Homemade varieties are best. Mix your oil with vinegar as a base then spice it up with garlic, onion, or poppy seeds.

Choose Your Seven Day Detox

Eating more fruits and vegetables is synonymous with cleansing the body of excess body fat and detoxing. The more fruits and vegetables you consume, the more vitamins you get, the easier it is for your body to detoxify itself, thus the less body fat you carry and the healthier you are. When this happens, you will experience a drastic reduction in inches around your waistline, and a high five from your partner.

Detox Level 1:   Making juices and smoothies with protein daily, plus eating whatever you want every 2-3 hours

Detox Level 2: Juices and smoothies daily, eating only fruits, vegetables, nuts, seeds, fish and eggs

Detox Level 3: Fresh natural juices, no smoothies! Eating only fruits, vegetables, nuts and seeds

Detox Level 4: Fresh natural juices only. No food at all

Did you notice how things seem to get a little harder as you go up in detox levels? Odds are, currently you are (at most) Level 1, consuming enough fruits and veggies to get your daily detox and reduce body fat. Take my advice, step it up for one week, and consider doing Level 3. Shoot for at least four days. When you're done with your juice cleanse, start adding more protein.

Start Your Juice Cleanse Detox

During the next 7 days, you are going to curb any craving you have for sugar, salt, and fats while building a new foundation for eating healthy. You will likely shed off some extra body fat while you're at it.

During this time, you are to consume no animal products and substitute in two juices each day, one in the morning and one in the afternoon. A cleanse promotes healing and detoxification within the body on a cellular level. It improves digestion and flushes out extra body fat and free radicals, while achieving higher energy levels through living foods. The irritants and toxins from your everyday diet are omitted and any remaining in the system begin to leave through the natural processes of elimination. Consuming no animal products allows energy normally used for digestion to supercharge your system with a flood of easy-to-assimilate vitamins and minerals. This cleanse will leave you addicted to only one thing: feeling amazing!

Sacrifice The Following	Eat As Much As You Want
Dairy Products	Salads
Meat & Poultry	Oil Dressings
Grain Products	Fruits & Vegetables
Cream-Based Soup	Berries & Nightshades
Preservatives	Nuts & Seeds
Artificial Flavorings	Chia & Flax Seeds
Caffeinated Drinks	Vegetable-Broth
Alcohol & Nicotine	Purified Water

The Only Thing You Need To Add To Your Juices

Essentially when you are juicing fruits and vegetables you are mainly getting carbohydrates and not much protein. Vegetarians know all about this. By adding in some natural sources of protein like chia seeds and flax seeds, you get the best of both worlds.

A.M. Juice – Add 2 tbsp. of Flax seeds and 2 tbsp. Chia seeds.

P.M. Juice – Add 2 tbsp. of Chia seeds, no Flax.

Chia Seeds – Your New Best Friend

These beauties are incredible! They are all-natural, have no Trans Fats and are 100% gluten free. Chia seeds are the richest whole food source of Omega-3s and Fiber in nature. They are a complete source of dietary protein, providing all the essential amino acids. Chia seeds will also help scrape through your digestive tract to remove any impurities and long-term plaque buildup. In 4 tablespoons of Chia seeds, you get 5 times more calcium than a glass of milk; 3 times more iron than a serving of spinach; 15 times more magnesium than a serving of broccoli; 2 times more potassium than a banana; and 3 times more antioxidants than a cup of blueberries.

Nature's Other Superfoods

Fruits

Cranberries
Strawberries
Raspberries
Blueberries
Grapefruit

Nuts & Seeds

Brazil Nuts
Walnuts
Sesame Seeds
Pumpkin Seeds
Cashews

Vegetables

Broccoli
Spinach
Cauliflower
Mushrooms
Onions

Super Foods

Honey
Garlic
Parsley
Lemon
Spices

Post Detox Food List

Now that you've had your "ceremonial sacrifice" with some contents from your kitchen, it's probably looking pretty empty. The list of ideas below aren't intended to be your only options. It's just to help you get started. Use these ingredients to cook up some recipes you like.

Fruits And Vegetables

Take a moment and stop to ask your grocer, "What's in season?" You'll be surprised by what you learn. Choose seasonal fruits and vegetables, and stick to local organically-grown produce. Whenever you can, head out to the farmers' market. Each fruit & veggie is specific in what vitamins and minerals it has in it. Organic produce is, on average, 40% more nutrient dense. Once you pick it from the tree, the nutrients start to die. Make sure to get your favorite leafy greens and mix it up from time to time. Just a quick word of advice: when you're starting to make healthy juices, try to keep the colors similar.

Extra-Lean Ground Beef

Search for the leanest ground beef you can find, and keep a couple of pounds on hand, frozen. The regular meat section will do, or again, head down to the local butcher shop or farmer's market to buy freshly-ground, grass-fed beef.

Chicken Breast

For now, the grain-fed store-bought will be fine. Cheaper brands hold a lot of water, and you'll know it because you'll see a strange white slime cooking off the sides when it comes out of the oven. As you start to increase your servings of protein, I suggest switching to organic because this usually is one of the biggest sources of toxins to our body. Think of it this way: your body can only be as healthy as the animal you eat, and the animal you eat is only as good as the plants it eats. Nowadays, most conventionally-fed animals eat only grain pellets. Opt for organic, and you know it's closer to the earth. For a change, pick up a whole chicken and toss it in a slow cooker. The bones and skins will give it a little more flavor then the same old boneless/skinless. If you don't have a slow-cooker, I suggest you get one. (Or, dust off the one you already have!)

Fresh Salmon

If you ever played sports back in the day, coaches used to say you should eat a huge plate of pasta the night before an event to boost your energy. Nowadays, they are saying healthy fats are the way to go. Wild Atlantic salmon, tuna, and tilapia are perfect for this. I suggest salmon because it has a great Omega-3 profile, and there is less likelihood of the high mercury levels and toxins sometimes found in farmed salmon. If you don't like fish, I recommend finding a high-quality Omega-3 supplement to provide you with the right balance of all 3 Poly, Mono, and Saturated fats- and don't worry about bad breath. There are many brands out there that have invested good money into making these things taste great, and don't have that the fishy aftertaste.

Cheese

Cheeses are fatty foods, so they should be eaten moderately. A serving of cheese should be around the size of a golf ball, and one serving per snack and meal will be enough. Opt for stronger-flavored varieties such as feta, goat, Havarti, mozzarella, aged white cheddar, and parmesan, so that you need less to give it a zing. These cheeses also typically have more protein and a better fat content. I recommend buying the partly skimmed mozzarella and feta.

Eggs
I prefer to buy Omega-3 eggs that come from chickens that have been fed an Omega-3 rich diet, this means 10-20% ground flax-seed. Typically, I recommend using one whole Omega-3 egg in each omelet together with egg whites to add additional protein.

Egg Whites
In addition to the whole Omega-3 omelets, I typically use about 1 cup to make protein pancakes, which are nothing but oats and high-quality protein. Purchase them in a carton, you can even find them for a good price at Costco. Try to go every other week to stock up on bulk items like this.

Foods To Horde And Pillage Over
If you have baking supplies, hordes of pasta, potato chips, crackers, cookies and other junk laying around, consider setting all of it ablaze, or carefully position a large garbage bin directly beneath the cupboard. With a quick side-motion, use your arm to plow these enemies into the abyss. You don't need personal training for this one! Stock up on some of the following foods. They're very conducive of clean eating.

Grains & Breads
White bread is broken down into sugar so quickly it might as well be sugar itself. If you're going to shop for these, always get whole grain or flat breads. Here are some of

the good-guys of the grain family: oat bran (whole, steel cut, rolled), whole flax seeds, quinoa, barley, and wheat bran. Notice that these don't require a lot of processing before they hit the shelf.

Nuts & Seeds

When you're looking at this self-serve nut section in the grocery store, think of it as being in the vitamin aisle at the drug store. Start packing these babies as part of your snacks or toss them in a smoothie. Don't overdo it on these. Remember, a serving of nuts & seeds is roughly the size of a golf ball. Walnuts, almonds, pecans, and cashews are some of the healthiest and best-tasting. Hit the bulk store every now and then to stock up. Remember, the oil content of these will dictate how long or short they will stay good. The higher the oil content, the quicker they will go bad. Quick tip: you can tell which are higher in oils by how soft or hard they are at room temperature. The higher the oil the softer they are and the quicker they go bad.

Canned Goods

Chickpeas, split peas, lentils and kidney beans are a great addition to your cupboard. You can choose to purchase the canned version although you should always go raw and fresh if you can. Toss some of these bad boys in your salad or crock pot to add protein and micro-nutrients vitamin mineral power. Not to mention, the fiber is great.

Dried Fruit

Be careful not to eat too many of these little devils! Most people are surprised to learn that 4-5 pieces have as many calories as an apple. You'll never eat 5 apples in one serving, but wouldn't think twice about putting back 20 of these. Dried fruit perfectly complements your oatmeal and salads. You can usually find a mix you like at the grocery stores. My personal healthy favorites include apricots, kiwis, pears, mango, bananas, and dates. Just be sure that you're not getting the highly-sweetened ones and watch out for hydrogenated oils, dyes, and flavors as additives. Remember, food manufacturers like to slip things in constantly. You will notice the sugars, oils, and other unhealthy chemicals in them when you look.

Oils

You have to consume fat to lose fat, and your brain is mainly built with fatty tissue. That is why it is so important to add in things like flax and Chia seeds into your detox program. Always get fresh oils, know which ones are going to be more stable with the temperature you're using to cook. They are used in salads, sauces, and for medium heat pan-frying. Look for "extra virgin" as it's the purest and most nutritious oil.

Spices

Healthy food doesn't have to taste brutal to be good for you! With this in mind, spices are your best friend. Salt is not bad when it's as close to nature as literally scraping it off the beach in Nova Scotia. (Himalayan sea salt is excellent!) Even a few spices can turn you into a master chef. There is a detailed list of spices on the following grocery list. A few basics to have on-hand are pepper, garlic, basil, oregano, chili powder, onion powder and cinnamon. Seasoning mixes like fajita mix are also good to have and take the guesswork out of the Mexican fiesta party you're having. Make sure you send an invitation for me to Optymal health Studios.

Your Post-Detox Grocery List

This list includes all the ingredients you will need for the recipes I use. Use the rest of ingredients to generate some other meal ideas, maybe dust off the crock pot and get out grandma's chili recipe. Definitely consider picking up the supplements. You don't need anything fancy.

MEAT & PROTEINS	OTHER STUFF
Extra Lean Ground Beef, 1-2lb	Salsa & Humus, 1 Jar Each
Chicken Breast, 1-2lb	Whole Wheat Fajita Wraps, 1 Bag
Extra Lean Turkey Breast, 1-2lb	Cooking Spray (Canola or Olive)
Salmon Fillet, 1lb	Steel Cut or Large Oats With Bran, ½ lb
Tofu or Soy Meat Substitute (If Vegetarian)	Whole Wheat Tostitos Chips, 1 bag
Omega-3 Eggs, 1 Dozen	Chia & Flax Seeds, 1 Bag Each
Egg Whites, 2 Cartons	Pecans or Walnuts, 1lb
Low Fat Feta & Low Fat Mozzarella Cheese	Quinoa Grain, 1lb
Cottage Cheese (1%Fat)	Extra Virgin olive Oil, Small Bottle
Organic Yogurt (0% Fat)	Balsamic Vinegar
Almond or Rice Milk	Diced Tomato & Paste, 2 Cans Each
FRUITS & VEGETABLES	Kidney Beans, 1-2 Cans
	Chick Peas, 1-2 Cans
Raw Arugula & Baby Spinach, 1lb Each	**SPICES**
Baby Carrots, 1 Bag	
Broccoli, 1 Bunch	Black Pepper & Sea Salt
Sweet Onion, 2 Medium	Cumin & Fajita Seasoning
Fresh Red Tomato's, 4 Large	Cinnamon & Spices You Like
Organic Cucumbers, 2 Large	Tupperware Containers For Lunches
Green Peppers, 4 Each	Protein Shaker Cup With Mixer Ball
Fresh Garlic, 1 Small Bunch	**SUPPLEMENTS**
In Season Apples & Oranges, 4 Each	
Lemons, 4 Each	High Quality Multi Vitamin, 1 Bottle
Organic Bananas, 1 Bunch	Vanilla Whey or Soy Protein, 2lb
Frozen Blueberries, 1 Bag	Omega Fish Oil Capsules, 1 Bottle

What To Take From This

After you've completed your cleanse, you will want to continue using all of these super foods, while slowly increasing your protein intake using healthy sources. A cleanse gives you a clean slate, so you will want to develop a healthy diet plan specific to your body type moving forward. Again, during your cleanse, you are essentially on a low-protein diet. Therefore, it is critical to incorporate as much Chia and Flax Seed to compensate as possible. In the next chapter, you'll find some of the best high-protein recipes I could gather for fat loss. Better yet, these recipes are so quick to prepare, they'll make your life much easier. Trust me! I've tried everything to get better results for my clients and myself. In fact, I probably know more about what doesn't work than anyone else. Still, knowing what doesn't work is the best way to figure out what does.

10

EAT CLEAN & TRAIN DIRTY

All foods can be divided and looked at in two different categories, these are called your Macronutrients (carbs, fats, proteins) and Micronutrients (vitamins and minerals). If you have ever taken economics, you have heard of the terms macro and micro, one means big the other means small.

Your macronutrients are your carbs, fats, and proteins. When you read a label, you will see calories at the top and then your macronutrients broken down underneath. All three of these combined will equal the amount of calories you get from eating that particular food. If you eat a Big Mac, it is a combination of macronutrients that will always equal out to a set amount of energy mesuared in calories. If you eat a cardboard box, it will be a compilation of carbs, fats, and proteins that will always equal out to, you guessed it, calories!

Calories are the unit of measurement that will gauge the amount of energy your body will get from eating a specific food. On the other side, the Micro level, you have your vitimins and minerals. You can recognize vitamins as your standard A's, B's and C's and a few others. Then, you have your minerals which are basically anything you would see on the periodic table, like Calcium, Potassium, or Magnesium. Your micronutrients are non energy-yielding, which means that you do not necessarily give you any energy but they help piece together the bigger picture in terms of your biochemistry.

This is Nutrition 101! If you can remember this you're set. You'll start understanding labels and the whole ball will start rolling in a much more informed direction. The one thing I want to establish at this point is this: any time I am talking about carbohydrates in the health bible, I am referring to carbs from fruits and vegetables.

Traditionally, people think of carbohydrates as what I would call "starchy carbs." These are things you want to limit because they often lead to inflammation and a spare tire/muffin top. This happens because most people are mildly allergic to gluten. If you want to know more about gluten, research it! I don't think giving you detailed facts about gluten will help you eat it less. They only thing I have to say is that if you remove gluten you will lose a few inches and start thinking more clearly. The biggest culprits I have found to cause inflammation are gluten, dairy, and some nuts and seeds depending on the person. The reason it depends on the person is that everyone's body is different, and almost everyone will be mildly allergic to certain things based on their genetic make-up and the environment they grew up in. Think of it this way, if someone is badly allergic to peanuts, their neck will swell up and they'll need an Epipen. This is called a hypoallergenic effect. It's possible that you are ingesting things that you are mildly allergic to you everyday. You just don't know it yet because you've lived with it for so long. This is yet another reason why you should keep a food journal. Interestingly enough, you can become more intolerant to these things as you get older. One thing I have always found to help, and one of the best tips I can give you, is that if you're a woman over 40, cut out gluten altogether.

From my years of experience as a certified nutrition coach, one critical point stands out: the reason it's hard to change habits is usually because of our self-gratifying urge to do the things that will not be good for us in the future. But once it goes south, we will spend everything we have, financially and emotionally, to get it back.

You should give yourself some credit for getting this far and taking these first steps. They're always the hardest ones, even when we know better. If you're anything like most people I talk to on a daily basis, you're probably searching for a realistic and permanent solution to your fat loss problems. Don't waste time on quick fixes or losing any more self-esteem. I am on a mission to revolutionize the fitness industry by dispelling the myths of the past with the following information. This stuff really works when you can educate yourself with it and apply it to your daily life.

How Much Food Should You Eat?

People know that if you overeat you will gain weight, however people often don't realize that if you under-eat, your body will store every gram of fat and calories you ingest. The following charts explain the calories to weight ratio.

FEMALE CALORIE LEVELS				
Weight	No Activity	Low Activity	Active	Very Active
100	1200	1400	1600	1700
110	1200	1500	1600	1700
120	1200	1600	1700	1800
130	1300	1600	1700	1800
140	1400	1700	1800	1900
150	1500	1700	1800	1900
160	1600	1700	1900	2000
170	1700	1800	1900	2000
180	1800	1800	1900	2000
190	1900	2000	2000	2000
200	1900	2000	2000	2000
200+	2000	2000	2000	2000
Based on the resting energy expenditures of 795+7.18 (kg) women (Source: Owens, 1986 American Journal of Clinical Nutrition)				
Formula for exact calorie level = (665.10 + (9.56 x weight in kg) + (1.85 x age in years)) + 200				

MALE CALORIE LEVELS				
Weight	No Activity	Low Activity	Active	Very Active
120	1500	1900	2100	2200
130	1500	2000	2100	2200
140	1600	2000	2100	2300
150	1700	2100	2200	2400
160	1800	2100	2200	2400
170	1900	2200	2300	2400
180	1900	2200	2400	2500
190	2000	2200	2400	2600
200	2000	2300	2500	2600
200+	2100	2400	2600	2800
Based on resting energy expenditure of 879 + 10.2 (kg) men (source: Owens, 1986 American Journal Of Clinical Nutrition)				
Formula for exact calorie level = (66.47 + (13.75 x weight in kg) + (5.0 x height in cm) – (6.76 x age in years)) + 200				

From what I have learned in business, the numbers don't lie! Most personal trainers and nutritionists realize this and use this to build your problem and capitalize on it as much as possible. The facts are simple, what you eat fuels your body with energy on a microscopic level. Thus, if you eat a certain amount of energy or calories every day, you will eventually achieve the weight of that caloric level. Without monitoring your food intake, you have not given yourself a chance of getting to your goal because the allowed margins for error are so small. Without monitoring, there is no way of knowing whether or not you are over or under-eating for your goal weight. That's why I have found keeping a food journal to be so effective. You must be precise and consistent to achieve results, this is why experts are calling it a science and that is why a lot of people resort to menu plans.

Don't get obsessed with how many calories you're eating. What's important is that you consistently eat clean and come up with new meal ideas that are easy to cook. Time management is important and if it takes long to do, you likely won't be consistent with it in the long term. If you're having trouble coming up with meal ideas or tracking your calories or energy intake, e-mail me at rob@optymalhealthstudios.com and we'll brainstorm some ideas together. Essentially what ends up happening with this method is that you are always aiming high and falling short. Thus, you're under-eating in the long run and keeping your body fat levels the same.

Keep It Simple

Again, the more effective way is to use the Universal Law of Averages, by eating 200 calories over your goal one day, and 200 calories below the next. This factors in all the possible activity levels and hits your target on average over the course of a month more frequently. It's like drawing the actual target around your mark, instead of trying to hit a bull's eye every day. In simplicity, if I am 180 lbs and I want to be 200 lbs, there is no way that I am going to get there unless I eat for a 200 lb male. You can also do the same in reverse, if you are 160 lbs woman and you want to be 140 lbs woman, then you should eat like a 140 lbs woman and factor in your activity level and you will eventually get there. The key is to eat for your goal weight. The simplest formula that I have found for calculating the amount of calories you need is to take your goal weight and multiply it by ten. Rocket science, right? That particular calculation will give you the amount of calories that your body needs while at rest for your goal weight.

Eat for your goal weight…

Goal weight x 10 = How much energy you need.

Factor in activity level…

Add 1 to the multiplier for activity,

What about my carbs, fats and proteins?

This is where we get some confusion!

Body Builders vs Vegans

In my opinion, every diet known to man falls between these two schools of thought. You have the body builders on one side saying you need high-protein everything plus ten shakes a day and you have the vegans saying that you get all the protein you need from fruits and veggies and that man was not meant to be eating dead flesh (meat protein). Both sides have valid points and have interesting arguments, and both sides have pros and cons. Personally, I don't believe there is one particular answer, it depends on the person and what body type they have.

How Much Carbs, Fats And Protein Do You Need?

Everyone is born with a unique set of genetics. This will determine not just how we look, but how our body uses energy and what your metabolic rate is. Genetically, you need to feed your body the type of fuel it needs to achieve optimal performance. Food breaks down and metabolizes at different speeds as well. Carbohydrates metabolize much quicker than fats, and protein digests much slower in general. Different macronutrients (carbs, fats and proteins) digest at different speeds. Learning this will help you discover how to eat before and after your workouts. Now, let's talk about what's best for you.

There are three body types to consider, each linked to your body's natural speed of digestion into energy and its base metabolic rate. The notion of individuality is key! There can never be any one diet or product that works for everyone. We must all discover which formula works for our biochemical and cultural individuality. There is no "one-size-fits-all" approach. Therefore, to achieve optimal health, you must determine what is right for you. You can get a sense of what body type and metabolic rate you have through examination of the wrist and phalange bones and also by taking a very simple metabolic typing questionnaire which will categorize you into one of three different categories. A simple way to remember this is to

consider what kind of genes you have from your
ancestors. If your ancestor's cohabitated in an area of the
world where they had long winters and needed to hunt
for meat protein to survive, you're likely a protein type. If
your ancestors lived in an area where it wasn't necessary
to hunt because all of their food could come out of the
garden, let's make life easier and eat carbohydrates! The
body is like a motor and you have to put the right kind of
fuel into it for it to run smoothly. Nowadays most people
are mixed types, but it's still something to consider for
overall optimal health and performance.

Equator Carb Type / Ectomorph
- Carbs = 70% of Calories
- Fats = 10% of Calories
- Proteins = 20% of Calories

Mixed Type / Mesomorph
- Carbs = 40% of Calories
- Fats = 30% of Calories
- Proteins = 30% of Calories

Polar Protein Type / Endomorph
- Carbs = 35% of Calories
- Fats = 20% of Calories
- Proteins = 45% of Calories

Once you know how much energy your body needs in the
form of calories, and you have the right macronutrient
ratios for your body type, you can start to do some math
to sort out how many grams of each macronutrients you
need. Dieticians and nutritonists will charge you hundreds
of dollars for this. You can do the math and save a ton of
money by using these charts. Think of it as your formula.

- **Carbohydrates:** 1 gram = 4 calories
- **Fats:** 1 gram = 9 calories
- **Proteins:** 1 gram = 4 calories

Remember, this information is simply a recommended guideline for after your detox. Be proactive and start reading labels more often so you can learn which foods are best for you. Figuring out your body type is quite simple, but if you're not sure which one you are, shoot me an email or call me and we can figure it out.

When To Eat

Meal timing is very important so I decided I would give you a breakdown of my own personal program. I work out in the mornings, and you should as well. This will spike your metabolism throughout the day, have you drinking more water, and help you sleep better by the time the evening comes around. Keep an open mind! This is just what I personally use and have seen work for a lot of people. Figure out what works best for you by following this outline and integrating the foods from the previous page. Just remember: eat everything in moderation and be consistent! The following is a great EZ meal break down I use during the week.

Meal 1 @ 9:00 AM/Pre-Workout
You want to start off with complex carbs such as 1 cup of Oatmeal (Add cinnamon for flavor) and maybe 1 Green Apple. Also add scoop of Protein between 30-40 grams + 1/2 L of water.

Workout @ 11:00 AM/Optymal Health Studios

If you're having trouble using this outline because your workout times are not in the AM, stop by the club during this time and I'll restructure something similar for you.

Meal 2 @ 12:10 PM/Recovery Shake
(This is The Most Important Meal After Breakfast)

Take 30-40 grams of Protein immediately after your workout in water or with a FRESH juice + 1/2 L of Water.

Meal 3 @ 1:30 PM / Post-Workout

After your workout, stick with simple carbs such as salad, juice, rice, pasta, or potatoes. They will dissolve faster than complex carbs. You need to replenish what you lost, and simple carbs break down faster. It's also the best time to eat red meat, because your metabolism is at its peak so it will break down easier.

Meal 4 @ 3:30 PM

Chicken, Yams, Potato, Broccoli, Cauliflower, and Avocado.

Meal 5 @ 7:00 PM

Fish should be your last heavy meal of the night due to its Omega fats. Also, 1 cup brown rice, any green veggie combined with half an avocado.

Meal 6 Before Bed

30 grams of whey isolate with a table spoon of all natural peanut butter. Drink at least 3-6 L of water per day!

Our body is made of nearly 70% water. When you're dehydrated, and most people are, your body will store more fat from the meals you eat. Plain and simple, we are a water species and we live on a water planet. Water flushes fat and it's a natural detoxifying agent.

How Much Protein Do You Need?

Some pro-vegetarian experts will have you believe that protein is somehow harmful and unnecessary. Don't get this idea stuck in your head, especially when they are referring to protein powders. I wrote a whole section for you on this later on. I find for health nuts, things like chicken and turkey are favorites because they don't have as much fat as red meats like beef or pork. I'm not saying that fat is bad. You just need to make sure you're not overdoing the fats when having protein with every meal.

Remember, we want the best of all possible worlds - the best health, body, and performance. It's pretty hard to have all three of these without adequate protein! You may be able to get enough protein having chicken with every meal, but I've found this very hard to do without supplementing in a smoothie or protein powder a few times per day. So make it easy on yourself and pick up some good quality protein. If you need advice, just ask.

Here's what you should aim for

- **Women:** 20-30 Grams of Protein a Meal – the equivalent of 1 palm sized portion of protein. Remember, protein is not limited to just breakfast, lunch and dinner. Every meal & snack, every 2-3 hours should contain protein.

- **Men:** 40-60 Grams of Protein a Meal – the equivalent of about 2 palm-sized portions.

By following the advice above, you'll not only ensure an adequate intake of protein, you will also maximally stimulate your metabolism, improve your muscle mass, recovery, and reduce your body fat.

Generally, you can only digest around 20-30 grams of protein per sitting. But, what constitutes a sitting? Is that every 2-3 hours? Personally, I think it is based on your body type, metabolism, and how much you exercise. I prefer to shoot a little higher so I have everything I need as my fitness level and metabolism changes.

Protein Supplements

Since opening up my first studio and juice bar, I've been approached by multiple nutrition companies to represent their products by offering it to my clients and in our recipes. If someone commits to one of my body transformation programs, I will literally offer them a guarantee to getting to their goal, and only have them using products that are conducive to the client getting there. For me to stand behind a company's products and actually say, "Yes, it's fine to take," it had better be good! After doing some due diligence and talking to many different people, I realized how confusing this industry really is. I could've started selling anything and making money off it, but I wanted to make sure that what we settled with was something that was simple and that would work for everyone.

Thinking about the bigger picture, there are 7 billion people on the planet that are registered, and probably another billion unregistered. If everyone is eating 3 nutritious meals a day, that equals to 24 billion meals that we need to find a way to provide. So how are we going to feed the planet in the future let alone now? Well we have already found one way, our farms are producing foods that are almost 100% genetically modified, and we don't even really know what damage GMOs can potentially do. Even simple things, like lettuce, are mostly hydroponically grown and isn't even grown in dirt. Doing some quick calculations, it takes about 45 heads of lettuce to match the nutrient content of one from about 20 years ago that was grown in the earth. It's basically water, fertilizer, and plant structure. I think the supplement industry will grow much larger over the next 50 years because we are going to need to make up for this lack of quality food and overabundance of people getting sick.

A low quality protein will make you sick if you are using it frequently over time, so pick a good one and know the labels are deceiving. A good protein supplement should have a good percentage of your day's calcium, and a balanced amount of all the vitamins and minerals that you need. It needs to have a solid amount of both soluble and non-soluble types of fiber. Without doing too much research around what is being hidden by the label, try this. Spray the sink down a bit so it's moist, then sprinkle a little protein powder on the surface and let it sit. I can tell you from doing this with so many products that if it's low in fiber, it will harden and require a strong set of nails to scrub off. Whatever happens here is what will happen in your stomach and digestive tract. It should also have three different sources of protein and minimal ingredients with names you cannot pronounce. Make sure it's not super high in sugars and check for the "other" names for sugar because, again, they will hide it well. It's all about building and maintaining lean muscle, which allows your metabolic rate to go up and you to burn fat even while you're sleeping. If you build lean muscle, you're burning fat 24 hours a day.

Now on to the biggest problem with these companies. They have to make their sales numbers and this often forces them to cut corners. They're not trying to kill you. In business, it's all about the bottom line!

Almost all of these protein supplement manufacturers are based in Florida because of how the industry started. The 2lb tub of protein usually retails for $45. That's normally the going rate, and has been for about 20 to 30 years or so. In order for these companies to get a 2lb container of whey protein out the factory door and to your kitchen, they have to keep the production costs to under $10/unit. That alone should make you wonder! Now, let's factor in the shipping costs, which averages $15, then $10 for the distributor, then another $10 for the retailer, leaving us with the going rate of $45!

In order to make your bottom line, and still have a product that's safe by government standards, it has to be 55% pure. So what these companies do is use a "cutting agent," or more commonly known as a "protein spike," their dirty little secret! What's even scarier is how many nutritionist know-it-alls at your local health food store don't know this.

The companies buy in bulk one single amino acid, usually Lucien, and fill the rest of the bottle with that, maybe adding in some additional synthetic vitamins to boost the quality. My mother is a pharmacist and ordering these powders is generally pretty easy, especially if you are a human biochemist or lab coat hanger. Buying these amino acids is like buying commodities, the prices go up and down month-to-month. Whatever is cheapest that season is the "flavor of the month" from my understanding. As long as its 55% pure branch chain amino acids, they can fill the rest of the container with what they have and boom! Now, the label can still say 100% protein because it's 100% pure branch chain of the 55%. Messed up, isn't it?

Personally, I prefer to buy products from multi-level marketing (M.L.M) companies because the distribution model is much different. They don't have to produce the product for under $10 to make up for all the other middle men. You M.L.M junkies are going to love me for this one.

Epic Juice Recipes

The difference between a juice and a smoothie is the yogurt, whey protein, or dairy product you add in to give it a smooth texture, hence "smoothie." All of these recipes are great for juice cleansing. You may want to add protein, depending on what level of detox you have chosen. After you're done with your cleanse, it's best to always add a high-quality protein supplement to help with digestion and assure you're getting what you need.

SPECIAL NOTE

Notice how we have at least one blended ingredient with each recipe? The only negative thing I have heard someone say about juicing is it removes the fiber. When you make your juices with a whole, blended ingredient, it really is the best of both worlds. The only downfall is you need to have both a blender and juicer to put these dandies together.

Wake Up Call
- **Blend:** Strawberries
- **Juice:** Apple, Beet, Pear, Lemon, Ginger

Berry Best
- **Blend:** Raspberries, Blackberries, Blueberries,
- **Juice:** Apple, Pear

Veggie Delight
- **Blend:** Cherries
- **Juice:** Cucumber, Carrot, and Beet

Cucumber Cooler
- **Blend:** Spinach
- **Juice:** Cucumber, Apple, and Pineapple

Watermelon Strawberry
- **Blend:** Strawberries, Raspberries
- **Juice:** Watermelon, Pear, Apple

Sure To Cure
- **Blend:** Mango, Peach
- **Juice:** Orange, Pineapple, Honeydew

Post Workout
- **Blend:** Blueberries, Cherries, Protein Powder
- **Juice:** Carrot, Oranges

Jungle Juice
- **Blend:** Spinach
- **Juice:** Celery, Cucumber, Honeydew

Fuzzy Peach
- **Blend:** Peach
- **Juice:** Apple, Carrot, Lemon

How To Choose A Juicer

After spending thousands of dollars and hundreds of hours trying to figure out the most efficient way to juice, I decided to help others in their quest for the most awesome juicer imaginable.

It all started in the founding days of my juice-cleansing program. I started looking at Canada's Food Guide and realized very quickly we needed to start replacing those massive suggested servings of starchy carbs with some fruit and veggie alkaline love.

As an experiment, I gathered enough fruits and veggies to take a good look at the amount needed for these suggested servings and realized it was a near impossible amount to consume.

After a few attempts, and therapeutic vomiting, I realized I could just juice the fruits and veggies together. That was my first experience with a juicer.

Realizing the potential, I started suggesting it to clients. They got great results, but for some reason they usually stopped after a few weeks. Unfortunately, the task of cleaning the juicer outweighed the results, even though it was good medicine.

The point I want to get across to you is this: you have to juice, and if you do it yourself, you will have to clean it up. So, before buying a juicer I suggest having an "emergency juice bar exit," in case you're lazy that day. Everyone has those days, don't worry. Even if you pick up a juicer after reading this and only use it a few times a week, it's better than nothing.

My first juicer was $127 and I got it at Bed, Bath, & Beyond. It lasted a long time considering all the juices I was making for my clients and myself.

Unfortunately, with small appliances, your chances of getting a "lemon" is high, and your chances of getting a cheaper juicer that lasts longer is just as good. Whatever you get, buy it from a solid appliance store with a great refund policy that doesn't require a receipt. Usually, the company that makes the returned product will reimburse the store you bought it. Just work on your negotiating skills and make sure you ask about that return policy.

The trick with a juicer is to get one that is easy to clean, and isn't expensive. Your best bet is to go with a combo appliance that comes with a juicer and a blender. Notice all the recipes in the health bible include a blended item alone with the rest of the ingredients that are juiced. You want to juice everything into the blender and add in the rest and hit start.

Having a dishwasher is helpful to clean everything except the screen, which will take a little scrubbing. If you have ever built anything before, you know jobs take twice as long without the right tools. Same is true when cleaning a juicer. If the spray nozzle on your kitchen sink has no pressure, the screen will take double the time to clean off.

In my experience, choosing a brand name for an appliance at the under $500 dollar mark doesn't make any difference. That's because they carry a celebrity's name or a well-known product name like VitaMix. VitaMix makes good products at the higher-end level.

Over the past few years, I've gotten a lot of experience in the department of buying juicers. Our juicer has gone down many times, and the industrial grade juicers range anywhere from $1,600 - $6,400 depending on what volume of juicing you're doing. These bad boys have motors measured in horsepower and juicing rates counted in gallons per hour. Recently, a company asked me if I wanted them to send a Swiss man down to my juice bar for a demo. Yes, he was coming from Switzerland and their products were over the $5000 mark. I had to tell him, "I need a juicer, not a Swiss missile guiding system!"

Redemption Smoothie Recipes

All shakes with (PW) mean post workout and (AT) means anytime. Take advantage of adding in supplements high in vitamins and nutrients. Adding a scoop of greens, or antioxidants can blast your smoothie to the moon and back! When making smoothies, get creative, shoot for the stars, and fall in the trees.

Banana Cream Smoothie (PW)

- 1 cup Water
- 1 cup Yogurt
- ½ Banana
- 1 tbsp Flax
- ½ cup Pecans or Walnuts
- 2 scoops Vanilla Protein

Almond Coconut Smoothie (AT)

- 1 cup Ice
- 1 cup Milk or Milk Substitute
- 1 tbsp Grated Coconut
- 1 tbsp Organic Cocoa
- 6 Almonds
- 1 scoop Vanilla Protein

Strawberry Banana Smoothie (PW)

- 1 cup Ice
- 1 cup Milk or Milk Substitute
- 1 medium Banana
- 1 cup Strawberries
- 1 scoop Vanilla Protein

Tigers Milk Smoothie (PW)

- 1 cup Tea
- 4 tbsp Yogurt
- 1 cup Frozen Berries
- 3 tbsp Steel-Cut Oats
- 1 serving Greens Plus (or any green supplement)
- 1 scoop Vanilla Protein

Nutty Sutty Smoothie (AT)

- 1 cup Milk or Milk Substitute
- ½ cup Ice
- ⅓ cup Low-Fat Cottage Cheese
- ½ oz. Almonds
- ½ oz. Walnuts
- 2 tbsp Flax
- 1 scoop Vanilla Protein

Chocolate Mint Smoothie (PW)

- ½ cup Water
- ½ cup Ice
- ⅓ cup Low-Fat Cottage Cheese
- ⅔ tbsp Mint Extract
- 1 tbsp Organic Cocoa
- 1 scoop Chocolate Protein

Chocolate Peanut Butter Smoothie (PW)

- ½ cup Ice
- 1 cup Milk or Milk Substitute
- ½ cup Low-Fat Cottage Cheese
- 2 tbsp Natural Peanut Butter
- 1 tbsp Organic Cocoa
- 1 scoop of Vanilla Protein

Morning Rush (AT)

- ½ cup Ice
- 1 cup Coffee
- 1 Banana
- 2 cups Milk or Milk Substitute
- 1 tbsp Organic Cocoa
- 2 scoops Vanilla Protein

Easy Fat-Loss Meals

Don't even try to say that you don't have time to prep your meals! If you want results, you have to put some time in. Take a few hours on a Sunday and pre-cook all your meals so it's quick and easy to put everything together. You have to stay several steps ahead of the game. The following are some of the cleanest and most balanced meals you can make!

Robby's Rockin' Oatmeal

Before going to bed, combine steel-cut oats, salt and 2 1/2 cups water in a non-stick pan, bring to a boil, remove from heat, and cover for the night. In the morning, bring to a boil again; add the oat bran, flax seeds, cinnamon, and the protein to sweeten the mix a little. Stir thoroughly, remove from heat, and add the berries.

- 1 cup Water
- ⅓ cup Steel-Cut Oats
- ⅓ cup Oat Bran
- 1 tbsp Flax Seeds
- ½ cup Blueberries (Frozen or Fresh)
- ½ tsp Cinnamon
- 1 scoop Vanilla Protein
- 1 dash Salt

Protein Pancakes

This recipe is my absolute favorite for Sunday mornings, or a late-night cheat meal when I'm feeling naughty. The measurements for this recipe are so easy, it's impossible to screw up. Grab a big bowl, throw in all the ingredients, and mix. Cook over medium heat, and enjoy! Go for a sugar free syrup, or make your own with Apple sauce and Natural peanut butter.

- 1 cup Whole Oats
- 1 cup Egg Whites
- ¼ cup Oat Bran
- ½ cup Blueberries or Banana
- 2 scoops Vanilla Protein
- 2 tsp Extra Virgin Olive Oil

Spinach and Feta Omelet
A simple North American breakfast classic. Stir-fry the chopped onions, mushrooms, peppers in a skillet coated with olive oil cooking spray on medium-high heat for 5 minutes, or until things begin to brown. Add the spinach and stir for about 30 seconds, just until the spinach becomes dark green and condensed. Add the beaten eggs. Wait a couple of minutes until you see bubbles starting to form around the edges of the eggs, then lift a portion of the eggs with a spatula, allowing the runny eggs on top to flow beneath the part that you lifted with the spatula. When the bottom of the omelet is solid again, flip the omelet. After flipping the omelet, add the feta of cheese to the top, still exposed in the skillet, and then fold the omelet over to cover the contents, then slide it onto a plate and enjoy!

- 3 Egg Whites, Plus 1 Omega- 3 Egg
- 1 handful Fresh Spinach, 2oz. Feta Cheese
- ⅓ chopped Onion, Red Peppers, and Mushrooms

Scrambled Green Eggs And Fake Ham

Stir-fry the chopped turkey, onions, and spinach in a skillet coated with cooking spray on medium-high heat for 3 minutes, or until the spinach becomes dark green and condensed. Add the eggs and cheese to the skillet and continue stirring for an additional 2 minutes, or until the eggs are cooked.

- 4 oz. chopped Turkey Bacon
- 1 slice Non-Fat Cheese
- 1 cup Egg Whites, Plus 1 Omega- 3 Egg, Beaten
- 1 handful Fresh Spinach
- ⅓ chopped Onion
- 2 tsp Extra Virgin Olive Oil

Post-Workout Oatmeal

Bring the water and salt to a boil in a saucepan, then turn the heat to low and add the oats. Cook for about 5 minutes, stirring regularly so that the oatmeal will not clump together. Add cinnamon, raisins and almonds, stir, cover the pan and turn off heat. Let sit for 5 minutes. Serve with milk and sweetener.

- 2 cups Water
- 1 cup Milk or Milk Substitute
- 1 cup Steel-Cut-Oats
- 1 dash Sea Salt
- ¼ tsp Cinnamon
- ¼ cup Raisins
- ¼ cup Sliced Almonds
- 1 tbsp Blackstrap Molasses

Chicken Quinoa

Cut the pre-roasted chicken breast into 1-inch cubes, then sauté together with the spinach in a large skillet coated with cooking spray. Cook just until warm, when spinach reduces and becomes limp. Reheat the steamed quinoa on the stove or in the microwave on a plate, and then top with the chicken and spinach. Add lemon juice and salt just before serving. Makes 1 large serving. Men may want to split it into two servings, and most women may want to split it into 4 beautiful servings for everyone to enjoy.

- 8 oz. Roasted Chicken Breast
- Steamed Quinoa Grain, From 1/2 Cup Dry
- Large Handful of Fresh Spinach Leaves
- 2 tbsp Lemon Juice Dash of Salt

Chicken And Chick Peas

In a large skillet, sauté the garlic in the olive oil over medium- high heat for a few seconds, then add the chicken and chopped onion. Stir-fry for 2 minutes until onions begin to brown. Add the remaining ingredients. Continue cooking and stirring for about 3 minutes, until the meal has a thick consistency. Makes 1 large serving. Men may want to split it into two servings; most women may want to split it into 4.

- 8 oz. Chopped Roasted Chicken Breast
- 2 cloves Chopped Garlic
- ½ Chopped Onion
- 1 can Chickpeas
- 2 tsp Extra Virgin Olive Oil

Fast Fajitas

One of my favorites because of the simplicity. Slice the chicken up with the onion and green pepper. Preheat your pan to medium-high and toss in the mix after spraying with olive oil. Sauté until chicken is fully cooked and spice it up with the cumin and fajita seasoning. Dish it out in a few wraps and add in the baby spinach with some salsa. Done! Pack a few for lunch tomorrow while you're at it.

- ½ lb Boneless/Skinless Chicken Breasts
- 1 large Sliced Onion
- 1 Green Bell Pepper
- 1 clove Minced Garlic
- ½ tsp ground cumin and fajita seasoning
- 3 tbsp Extra Virgin Olive Oil
- Baby Spinach
- Whole Wheat Fajita Wraps
- Salsa

Mediterranean Salad

Some people prefer to peel the cucumber first, but this is not necessary. Simply chop the cucumber and tomato into small cubes, then toss with the olive oil, salt, and feta if you like. Serve chilled. Makes 2 servings.

- 1 Sliced Cucumber
- 2 Chopped Tomatoes
- 2 cubes of Crumbled Feta
- 2 tsp Extra Virgin Olive Oil

Stuffed Peppers

Amazing for dinner or lunch the next day, these babies are loaded with flavor and make a great dinner or lunch for the next day. Not all stuffed peppers are cooked with rice, try using Quinoa or even crush up some of the tortilla chips if you're punched for time.

Heat oven to 400° and spray a little olive oil in a medium sized pan. Heat on medium, add onion, garlic and cumin. Cook for about 2 minutes and add ground turkey or chicken. Season with salt, garlic powder (if you want), and brown meat until meat is completely cooked through. Stir in cooked quinoa or tortilla chips to the mix. Cut the top of the peppers, and remove the seeds. Place in a baking dish and spoon feed the mixture into each pepper and cover the top with a little partly skimmed low fat mozzarella or Feta cheese. Cover tight with aluminum foil and bake for about 35 minutes.

- 1lb lean ground turkey or chicken
- 1 clove Minced Garlic
- ½ chopped onion
- 1 tsp cumin powder
- 3 large green bell peppers
- 1 ½ cups cooked rice
- ¼ cup of cheese
- 2 tsp Extra Virgin Olive Oil

Dirty 30 Chili

It's only dirty because it's ready in 30! In a large pot heat the oil over medium-high and add the onions and garlic.

Season with salt and pepper if you like, and cook stirring for about 5 minutes. Add tomato paste, chili powder, and cinnamon, then cook the mixture for 5 minutes. Add beef and cook for 5 minutes breaking it up until no longer pink. Add diced tomatoes and beans. Bring to a boil, and reduce to a rapid simmer. Cook over medium heat until chili has thickened slightly and beans are tender, about 5 minutes. Sprinkle with mozzarella or feta cheese if you like.

- 3 medium Chopped Onions
- 6 cloves Chopped Garlic
- 1 dash Salt and Pepper
- 1 can Tomato Paste (6 oz.)
- 3 tbsp Chili Powder
- ½ tsp Ground Cinnamon
- 2 lbs Ground Beef, Chicken or Turkey
- 3 cans Diced Tomatoes in Juice (14 oz. each)
- 2 cans kidney beans, drained (14.5 oz. each)
- Mozzarella or Feta cheese (optional)
- 1 tbsp Extra Virgin Olive Oil

3 Minute Generation X-Girl Guacamole

Combine all ingredients in a blender and blend for 1 minute. Alternatively, you can mash the avocado with a potato masher or fork and then add the rest of the ingredients. Serve these baby's with carrots, celery and cucumber dippers.

- 1 Medium Ripe Avocado and Diced Tomato
- 1 tbsp Lemon or Lime Juice, Salt and Pepper

Sweet Potato Parables

Fill the bottom of a steamer with 2 inches of water. While steam is building up press or chop garlic and let sit for at least 5 minutes. Cut potatoes in half and cut into 1/2" slices. You do not need to peel if they are organic. Steam sweet potatoes for no more than 7 minutes. Transfer to a bowl. For more flavor, toss sweet potatoes with the remaining ingredients and any of the optional ingredients you desire while they are still hot.

- 1 lb Diced Sweet Potatoes
- 2 cloves Chopped Garlic
- 1 dash Sea Salt & Pepper
- 2 tbsp Ground Pumpkin Seeds
- 2 tbsp Chopped Rosemary
- 3 tbsp Extra Virgin Olive Oil

Pecan Crusted Salmon

Wash the salmon fillet and pat it dry with a paper towel. Combine the olive oil, pecan meal, salt and pepper, and distribute the mixture over a clean plate, and then press both sides of the salmon into the mixture. Heat a nonstick skillet on medium-high heat, and sear each side of the fillets for 4 minutes. While the salmon is cooking, steam the spinach in a pot with a tight fitting lid over 1-inch of boiling water. Drain, and toss with the unsalted butter. Men may want to split it into two servings, and woman may want to split into 4.

- 10 oz. De-Skinned Salmon Fillet
- 2 tbsp Crushed Pecan Meal

- 1 dash Salt and Pepper
- 2 handfuls Raw Spinach and
- 1 tsp Butter or Butter Substitute
- 1 tsp Extra Virgin Olive Oil

Easy Cheesy Meat Loaf

Preheat the oven to 350°. In a skillet, sauté the onion, celery, garlic, and parsley in the oil over moderate heat until softened but not browned. With a slotted spoon, transfer the vegetables to a large bowl. Add all remaining ingredients, except cheese, to the vegetables. Mix well with your hands. Transfer half the mixture to a 9- by 5-inch loaf pan. Place mozzarella slices on top, then cover with the rest of the meat mixture. Bake for 75 to 80 minutes or until a meat thermometer reads 170°.

- ¾ cup Finely-Chopped Onion
- ½ cup Finely-Chopped Celery
- 2 tsp Minced Garlic
- ½ cup Minced Italian Parsley
- 1 tsp Sea Salt
- ¼ tsp Pepper
- 1¾ tsp Chili Powder and Cumin cup Salsa
- 2 Eggs
- 1½ pounds Lean Ground Beef or Turkey
- ¾ cup Breadcrumbs
- ¼ pound Sliced Mozzarella Cheese
- 2 tsp Extra Virgin Olive Oil

Cheesy Chicken Broccoli Soup

In a large pot, sauté the onions and mushroom in the

olive oil until tender. Add the Chicken Stock and bring to a boil. Once boiling, at the noodles, boil for 5 minutes. Add the diced chicken and broccoli and let cook for 5 minutes. Remove from heat and add the skim milk and cheese. Stir to melt the cheese and serve.

- 6 cups Chicken Stock
- 3 cups Milk or Milk Substitute
- 1 cup Finely-Chopped Onion
- 1 cup Sliced Mushrooms
- 1 (10z Pkg) No Yolks Wide Egg Noodles
- 1 Cup Diced Cooked Chicken (White Meat Only)
- 1 head Chopped Broccoli (or Asparagus)
- 1 pkg Low-Fat Cheddar Cheese
- 3 tsp Extra Virgin Olive Oil

Bean Dip

Place all ingredients into Crockpot cook until ingredients simmer down and form a paste like dip (approximately 1 hour). Enjoy ☺

- 8oz. can Organic Red Kidney Beans
- 8oz. can Organic Black Beans
- 8oz. can Organic White Beans
- 8oz. can Organic Yellow Corn
- ½ Finely-Chopped Green Pepper
- ½ Finely-Chopped Red Pepper
- ½ Finely-Chopped Yellow Pepper
- ½ Finely-Chopped Yellow or Purple Onion
- 1 clove Minced Garlic
- The following spices (to taste):

- Cayenne pepper
- Dash of Black Pepper and Chili powder
- Hot Sauce

Beef Barley Soup

Trim fat from meat; cut meat into 1/2-inch cubes. In a Dutch oven combine meat, water, celery, mushrooms, carrots, onion, salt, rosemary, pepper, and garlic. Bring to boiling; reduce heat. Cover for 1 to 1&1/4 hours or till meat is tender. If necessary, skim fat. Stir in tomato paste and barley. Return to boiling; reduce heat. Cover and simmer about 10 minutes or till barley is done.

- 1½ lb Boneless Beef Chuck
- 6 cups Water
- 1½ cups Sliced Celery
- 1½ cups Sliced Fresh Mushrooms
- 1 cup Sliced Carrots
- 1 cup Chopped Onion
- 1 tsp Sea Salt
- 1 tsp Crushed Dried Rosemary
- ½ tsp Pepper
- 1 clove Minced Garlic
- 1 (6oz.) can Tomato Paste
- ½ cup Quick-Cooking Barley

Pasta and Tuna Salad

Cook pasta according to package directions, but eliminate salt. About 7 minutes before pasta is done, add green beans to pot. Remove pot from heat and add onion.

Drain in colander and rinse under cold water. Drain again. While pasta mixture is draining, combine dressing, parsley, and chopped basil in large serving bowl. Mix well. Add pasta mixture to dressing mixture. Add tomatoes and tuna. Toss to coat. Garnish with basil sprigs and serve.

- 8oz. Tricolor Corkscrew Pasta
- 16oz. Green Beans, Trimmed and Cut into 2-Inch Pieces
- 1 Thinly Sliced Medium Red Onion (about 1 cup)
- ⅔ cup Reduced-Fat Italian Salad Dressing
- ¼ cup Chopped Fresh Parsley
- ¼ cup Chopped Fresh Basil
- 1 cup Halved Cherry Tomatoes
- 2 (6⅛oz.) cans Tuna Packed in Water, Drained and Flaked.
- Fresh Basil Sprigs for Garnish

Southwest Chicken

May seem like some work at first, I assure you it's not! In a large skillet combine tomato sauce, orange juice, onion, raisins, pimiento, oregano, chili powder, garlic, and hot pepper sauce. Bring to boiling; reduce heat. Cover and simmer for 5 minutes. Stir in chicken; return to boiling. Cover and simmer 12 to 15 minutes more or till chicken is tender and no longer pink. Meanwhile combine cornstarch and water. Stir into skillet. Cook and stir till thickened and bubbly. Cook and stir 2 minutes more. Toss parsley with rice. Serve chicken mixture over rice or Quinoa if you have looking for a starch from South of the boarder.

- 1 (8oz.) can Tomato Sauce
- ½ cup Orange Juice
- ½ cup Finely-Chopped Onion
- 2 tbsp Raisins
- 2 tbsp Chopped Pimiento
- ½ tsp Crushed Dried Oregano and Chili Powder
- 1 clove Minced Garlic
- 12oz. Boned Skinless Chicken Breast Halves, Cut into 1-Inch Pieces
- 2 tsp Cornstarch
- 1 tbsp Water and Hot Sauce
- ¼ cup Snipped Parsley
- 3 cups Hot Cooked Rice or Quinoa

Spicy Garlic Shrimp

Thaw shrimp, if frozen. Peel and de-vein shrimp; cut in half lengthwise. Set aside. In a mixing bowl stir together water, ketchup, soy sauce, rice wine or dry sherry, cornstarch, honey, crushed red pepper, and ground ginger, if using. Set aside. In a large skillet or wok stir-fry green onions, garlic, and fresh grated gingerroot, if using, in hot oil for 30 seconds. Add shrimp. Stir-fry 2 to 3 minutes or till shrimp turn pink; push to sides of skillet or wok. Stir ketchup mixture; stir into center of skillet. Cook and stir till thickened and bubbly. Cook and stir 2 minutes more. Stir sauce a Eat Clean & Train Dirty If desired, serve with hot cooked rice and pea pods.

- 1 lb Fresh or Frozen Shrimp
- 1 tbsp Water
- 2 tbsp Ketchup

- 1 tbsp Liquid Aminos (Soy Sauce)
- 2 tbsp Dry Sherry or Rice Wine
- 3 tsp Cornstarch
- 1 tsp Honey
- ½ tsp Crushed Red Pepper
- I tsp Grated Ginger
- ½ cup Sliced Green Onions
- 4 cloves Minced Garlic
- 1 tbsp Extra Virgin Olive Oil
- Hot, Cooked Rice (Optional)
- Fresh or Frozen Pea Pods (Optional)

Salsa Tuna Wrap

Mix the following in a small bowl or container for easy storage in a lunch bag. Spread the mixture in a wrap, whole grain bread or lettuce leaf.

- 1 can of Water-Packed Tuna
- 1-2 tbsp of Chunky salsa
- 1 dash Pepper

Shanghai Beef or Chicken Stir-Fry

Heat a large nonstick skillet wiped with olive oil on medium-high heat. Add meat and garlic; stir-fry for 2 minutes. Add vegetables, dressing and soy sauce; stir-fry an additional 3 minutes or until everything is cooked through. Spoon rice into serving platter; top with meat mixture.

- 1lb (500 Grams) Boneless Beef Sirloin Steak (or 3

Large Chicken Breasts), Cut Into Thin Strips.
- 2 tsp Minced Garlic
- 1 package of Frozen Stir-Fry Vegetables (750 grams)
- ½ cup of Asian Sesame Dressing
- ¼ cup of Liquid Aminos (Soy Sauce)
- 3 cups of Hot, Cooked Long-Grain Brown Rice

Turkey Meatballs

Mix everything together in a large bowl, then separate into 2 inch meatballs and place on a cooking sheet coated with olive oil. Bake at 375 F for 30 minutes or until a toothpick inserted comes out clean. For crispy meatballs, after 25 minutes put the meatballs on broiler for an additional 5-7 minutes keeping your eye on them.

- 1lb Ground Turkey
- ½ cup Ground Flax Seeds
- ¼ cup Bran
- ½ Finely Chopped Onion
- 4 cloves Chopped Garlic
- 1 Omega 3 Egg Plus 3 Egg Whites
- 1 dash Sea Salt & Pepper

Peppered Beef and Veggies

Cook spaghetti according to package directions. Drain well and keep warm. Meanwhile, for sauce, in a small bowl stir together water, soy sauce, cornstarch, green and red pepper, Set aside. Spray a cold wok or a large skillet with nonstick spray coating. Heat over medium-high heat. Add garlic and stir-fry for 1 minute. Add pea pods and green or red pepper, stir-fry 1 minute. Add mushrooms; stir-fry 1 to 2 minutes more or until vegetables are tender. Remove from wok. Add oil to wok. Stir-fry beef in hot oil for 3 to 4 minutes or until done. Push beef to side of wok. Stir sauce and pour into the center of the wok. Cook and stir until thickened and bubbly. Return vegetables to wok; cook and stir all ingredients 1 minute. Toss with spaghetti.

- 4oz Gluten Free Spaghetti
- ½ cup Water
- ¼ cup Low-Sodium Soy Sauce
- 2 tsp Cornstarch
- ½ tsp Pepper
- ½ tsp Ground Red Pepper
- 1 clove Minced Garlic
- 1 cup Fresh or Frozen Pea Pods
- ½ cup Chopped Green Pepper
- ¼ cup Chopped Sweet Red Pepper
- 1 cup Sliced Mushrooms1 tbsp Virgin Olive Oil
- ¾ lb. Lean Beef Cut Into Bite-Size Strips

Big Haus Burritos

Wrap tortillas in foil. Heat in a 350 degree oven for 10 minutes to soften. Meanwhile, for filling, cook ground beef and onion until meat is brown and onion is tender. Drain, stir in black beans, un-drained tomatoes, and chili powder. Simmer uncovered, 5 minutes or to desired consistency. Reserve ¼ cup filling; set aside. Spoon ¼ of the remaining filling onto each tortilla just below center. Fold bottom edge of tortilla up and over filling. Fold opposite sides of tortilla in, just till the meet. Roll up from the bottom. Top with some of the reserved filling. Sprinkle with green onion.

- 4 10-inch Whole Wheat Tortillas
- ½ lb. Extra Lean Ground Beef
- 1 cup Chopped Onion
- 1 (10oz.) can Tomatoes
- 1 tsp Chili Powder
- 1 chopped Green Onion

Sutton Stir-Fry

Bring out a marvelous Asian wok or pan, only fit for the finest of Royal families. Drizzle oil into your wok or frying pan, slice boneless chicken or lean beef into strips, sprinkle black pepper, onion and garlic powder, brown the meat & drain grease. Chop green peppers, red peppers, onions, broccoli, carrot slices, cauliflower or other veggies as desired. Add to pan and cover. Add some water if the pan is dry. You can also use chicken or beef stock or stir-fry sauce for more flavor (be careful of extra calories and sodium content). Simmer until veggies are lightly steamed. Enjoy with whole grain rice!

- 1lb Boneless Chicken Breast or Lean Beef
- 1 Green Pe
- 1 Red Pepper
- 1 Onion
- Broccoli & Cauliflower
- Carrot Slices

- Black Pepper
- Onion & Garlic Powder
- Extra Virgin Olive Oil

Vegetarian Chilly

Vegetarians taste better! Especially with a little Chilly on the side. Use one package of vegetarian burger mix and cook through. This should be roughly equal to the amount you would use for four burgers. Chop the onions, green peppers and garlic. Combine the rest of the ingredients in a large pot. Crumble the burger and add to the chili sauce. Simmer away for thirty minutes.

- 4 Large Egg Whites
- 16oz Tofu Burger Mix
- 1 cup Chopped Onion
- 1 cup Chopped Green Pepper Bell Peppers!
- ½ cup Sliced Carrots
- 3 cloves Garlic
- 16oz Crushed Canned Tomatoes
- 16oz Tomato Sauce
- 16oz can of Kidney Beans
- 1 tbsp Chili Powder
- 1 dash of Cumin
- 1 dash Cayenne Pepper

Raspberry Almond Parfait

Blend yogurt, honey and almond extract in a small mixing bowl with a whisk until the honey is incorporated and the mixture is smooth. Divide the yogurt mixture into two dessert dishes. Place the raspberries in one layer on top and garnish with the sliced almonds and dark chocolate.

- 8oz Low-Fat Vanilla Soy Yogurt
- ½ tsp Almond Extract
- 2 tbsp Honey
- 1 pint Raspberries
- 1 tbsp Sliced Almonds
- Optional: Grated Dark Chocolate

Healthy Chocolate Pudding

My absolute favorite post workout snack pack. Toss everything into a high powered blender and blend on high for approximately 4 min, beauty!

- 2 cups of Trail Mix or Nuts of Choice
- 1 Banana
- ⅓ cup Chia Seeds
- 1½ cups Milk or Milk Substitute
- 2 scoops of Vanilla Protein

What To Take From This

This chapter is loaded with info that's taken my personal training to the next level. You'll notice this chapter often refers to fitness, and that's where we're going next. Now that you have all the recipes that I've used to bring my fitness goals to reality, it's time to take on the myths, and approach fat loss scientifically.

11

SCIENTIFIC FAT LOSS

The big box gyms and nutrition companies are stealing your money and abusing your trust in the name of product and membership profits. The real truth is, most of the products and services being sold are worthless to you. Obviously, to them they are incredibly valuable because they're raking in huge profits at your expense. Your health is the most valuable asset you have. The following are the 3 biggest fat loss myths people fall into believing.

Myth #1 "Dieting Will Eliminate Body Fat"

Ask yourself first, what is a diet? A diet is a way of eating and I put my clients on new diets all the time. The traditional word "dieting" refers to denying your body the essential nutrients and calories it needs to function efficiently. Calories are the unit of measurement we use to calculate the amount of energy available after eating something. In the beginning of a diet you WILL lose weight, but it won't be body fat, it will be body water and lean muscle tissue. This is the exact OPPOSITE of what you want to do. This means you actually want to increase body water and lean muscle to flush out body fat and keep it off permanently.

Most of the people I've worked with were "dieters" before coming to see me and everyone knows that you can't sustain not eating indefinitely. Your body screams out for nourishment and eventually you will be running for high calorie foods. This is called the rebound effect and is where the term "yo-yo diet" comes from. When this happens you will always regain the body fat you lost – and then some! The biggest problem is during your diet your body cannibalized the lean muscle as fuel. After the diet, your regained weight is not in the form of lean muscle plus some fat – it comes back almost exclusively as fat! When you dramatically reduce your caloric intake, your body shifts into a protective mode by slowing your metabolism down and holding onto every gram of fat it can. See, your body intuitively knows that fat is an important source of energy, so it wants to hold onto it and burn muscle instead. To permanently reduce your body fat you've got to burn more calories through exercise and increase your metabolism by building lean muscle and eating healthy foods. Keep it simple!

All you need is a routine exercise program and proper macronutrient ratio adaptations to transform your body permanently. That's it! Balance your macronutrients, meaning to eat the right amount of carbs, fats, and proteins, at the right intervals and take your workouts very seriously. Don't miss a single one! Even if you don't exercise (but I recommend you do), just eating 5 - 6 small, high quality meals each day will substantially increase your metabolism – and you'll burn more body fat.

Myth #2 "Aerobic Exercise Will Burn Body Fat"

I've seen women who use their membership spending 5 days a week, 30 minutes at a time on the treadmill or stair climber and they don't lose weight at all! I know men who run 5km a day, who have no muscle but tons of jelly rolls around their waists. You've been lead to believe that if you want to lose body fat, all you have to do is regular cardio. I want to tell you about something called the Kreb Cycle. The Kreb Cycle means that in order for your body to shift into a fat burning state, there are 52 chemical reactions that need to take place. Even if you're fit, it takes 27 minutes before you can get there. If you use your membership to do a half hour of cardio, good job! You've burnt fat for 3 minutes! That being said, shorter more intense intervals of aerobic activity have been found to be extremely effective, but you must be able to monitor and control the intensity to maximize the number of calories you burn. If cardio is not supplemented with resistance training (lifting weights) to at least maintain lean muscle, you cannot effectively accelerate the fat loss process. Therefore, a combination of properly monitored cardiovascular exercise and resistance training enables you to rapidly burn the maximum amount of fat, in the shortest period of time.

SPECIAL NOTE

This may sound strange to you, it's fact not fiction! With the proper fitness and nutrition system in place, you can quickly burn fat and tone up in as little as 38 minutes per day. If you can exercise in the privacy of your own home in weeks you can dramatically transform your body.

Myth #3 "Resistance Training Doesn't Burn Fat"

Nothing could be farther from the truth! Muscle tissue is metabolically active, meaning the more you have, the more energy your body is infused with. The more lean muscle you have, the more fat you burn – even when you're at rest. Fat does not use energy – it is used as a powerful source of energy once it's burned. Muscle uses energy, lots of it! The more lean muscle you have, the more fat you're burning all day long! Building lean muscle is the #1 most effective way to keep body fat off permanently. Fat is simply a reserve tank fuel source for the body and most people have way more than they need in that reserve tank.

You see, that's really the ultimate fat loss secret! However, you can only exercise so much in a given week without messing up all the other complex systems of the body. The real secret is how metabolically active your body is the other 90% of the time. People with more lean muscle burn fat at a much greater rate than do those with less lean muscle. That doesn't mean you have to look like Brad or Angelina to be an efficient fat-burning machine. You do have to at least maintain, and preferably increase, your lean muscle tissue.

SPECIAL NOTE

Women will not become "bulky" or "muscle-bound" by incorporating resistance training into their exercise routine. In fact, just the opposite is true! Lean muscle is more compact and firmer than fat. Resistance training will make women smaller, firmer and sexier. Women are not genetically predisposed to adding muscle "mass." Men, on the other hand, will gain mass and see exciting muscle growth through the proper use of nutrition and resistance training. If you feel this way, I can tell you it's an illusion.

Exposed Secrets From The Pros

Commit to a workable plan of action! The big corporations are stealing your money and want you to believe that pills or gym memberships will solve all your fat loss problems. This is counter-intuitive and should insult your common sense now that you know better. But why are people still tossing their money away? Is it because they don't have the mental capacity to truly understand what is best for them? The real "secret" is quite simple and I'll distill it for you right here: eat 5 to 6 small healthy meals per day and perform a combination of aerobic and resistance training exercise for 40 to 60 minutes 3 times a week. Take out your calendar right now and mark off three days each week for the next 12 weeks when you will commit to exercising. Then do it! Your consistent commitment will bring you the results you want.

Learn from someone who has done it before! A coach is an experienced and trusted trainer or teacher and almost every self-help book ever written talks about the importance of having a coach/mentor. It's unavoidable that you will come up against hard times on your path to getting in shape. A coach will educate, guide, motivate and support you – so you can easily and rapidly overcome the things that get in the way. A coach is critical to systemizing your exercise program for maximum results and assisting you in heightening your motivation and strengthening your commitment. A coach becomes your "objective feedback system" helping you see, understand, and correct the problems that are interfering with your progress. Exercise and nutrition are bona-fide sciences and learning everything you need to know on your own can take years of struggle.

Always plan to progress to the next level! Have you ever met someone who says they workout week after week, month after month and haven't seemed to have changed at all? Believe me, doing the same workout over and over without any program to help you progress to the next level will actually decrease your fitness and cause a plateau. You must learn how to progressively improve and fine-tune your efforts for maximum fat loss results in minimum time. Considering everything else you may have spent time and money on, in the past, planning out every workout will give you the quick fix results you have been looking for.

The biggest secret is accountability! This is why workout buddies can work so well in the beginning. The only problem is who is going to stray from the program first? In a recent study at Virginia Polytechnic University, researchers divided people starting a walking program into two groups. Every week, each individual in one group got a phone call asking how their exercise program was coming along, the other group got no calls at all. At the end of 24 weeks, 45% of the individuals who got the phone calls were still walking compared to just 2% who did not receive calls. The results show that weekly accountability increases the likelihood of sticking to your exercise program by 2200%!

The key point is simple: when you have someone to hold

you accountable to a healthy 1.6 pounds of fat loss each week, you will make it happen. I have some clients that just come in for nutritional program design and others that even take their stats at home and call it in. Either way can work. However, those who don't have an accountability system usually fail.

What you've just read is some of the most valuable information you will ever hear on how to lose body fat and keep it off permanently. As I said earlier, understanding how the body works is critical to making healthier choices. That being said, intellectually understanding what should be done and actually doing it are two different things. I have discovered that the ultimate secret to getting the results you want is finding a coach who understands your needs and provides you with an effective fat loss and exercise program front lines…but most of all, a coach who holds you accountable!

At least now you know the truth. There is no quick fix, no special pill, and no New Year's membership that is going to suddenly make you fit. The multi-million dollar corporation's mainstream advertisements know how to push your emotional buttons and you are bombarded by them daily. They know how to get you to pull out your credit card. It's not the pill, powder, fancy gym membership, or the expensive equipment that will get you healthy and fit. The only thing that works is commitment to a healthy diet and regular exercise. You've got to piece together the information in this chapter and take action! There is only one way to cultivate your motivation and internalize your commitment: you must personally experience fitness results and start exercising! If you're honest with yourself and recognize that diet and proper exercise are the only ways to achieve the results you want, then you are ready to make a permanent lifestyle change.

Through my experience, education and extensive study, I have developed an approach to exercise that has enabled many average individuals to achieve amazing fat loss, health, and fitness results. It's a program that will support you in becoming laser-focused on the results you want, empower you to accept responsibility for making effective exercise part of your lifestyle, and provide you with the tools you need to reach your fitness goals. All it requires is 3% of your time. Just three percent! If you want to chat, just shoot me over an quick "what's up" email to rob@optymalhealthstudios.com and we can talk.

90 Workouts In 90 Days Will Change Everything

Let's start from the top: a workout does not have to be an hour and a half long session at the gym with free-weights. Take the stairs, move the blood, simply sweat is all I'm saying. You don't need a gym membership or expensive home fitness equipment. You don't need fad diets or medication. You don't need videotapes, books, or manuals. You don't need anything but guidance, support, motivation, and accountability. That's it! It's amazing how, by following a common-sense program, so many individuals have changed their lives from unhealthy and unhappy, to fit and ready to rock. I don't like the deception and misinformation that's being forced on us by the nutrition and fitness industries. It's sabotaging our self-esteem in the name of large profits. You can be absolutely certain that I am motivated by one thing and one thing only: educating and informing you about the only thing that really matters, results! So if you are open to results, and will accept what doctors have been saying for years, then I will show you the simplest way to do it. We are all mature adults. You've been around and lived probably longer than me. Being fit positively affects everything in your life: your health, your mood, your sex life, your financial success…everything! Make your body speak volumes about who you are.

Are You Certified?

The personal training industry in not regulated like massage therapy. How many great massages have you had from someone who isn't certified? This leads to a big pricing range and makes it a very lucrative business to be in if you're good. There is no governing body and no standards of practice except by the gym or person training. That's why it's so important to know the core values of the company under which you're training.

I've met average people that compete in fitness competitions who make amazing trainers, and people that have a kinesiology degrees who suck. I've met trainers overly certified and looking for more courses, but they have zero testimonials to their name. My general rule is to pick a good certifying course and only take another once you have gathered three testimonials from your current clients. You don't want to spend more on certifications then you make from training. That's Business Building 101 and, unfortunately, where most trainers drop the ball. The reality is, you can go online and take any random certification program, pay your $30, and it'll be in your inbox in 30 minutes. Yeah, before the end of this sentence you can be assured that I will be an ordained minister at www.ordainmenow.com.

You have to understand anatomy and how complex movement can actually be, if you are to become a personal trainer. Knowing the key areas like the center of gravity and the transverse abdominus is where I started after my first certification. A common phrase I teach my trainers is, "Don't Guess, Assess!" That's the key when they are choosing your exercises. I mean why couldn't your trainer just print off a program from the internet and pass it off as their own?

What matters to me is outlined in the back of the Health Bible under the "Where Do I Spend My Money?" section. I know what you're thinking, and no, I'm not trying to sell you personal training though a book. I wrote this as a guide to outline the most important daily workout duties all trainers must do. The biggest one, in my opinion, is empower you and not accept your excuses. You have to have someone you will be completely honest with and is willing to drop you as a client, if you're not open to small progressive changes.

Spinal Health

The more you know about the body, the more you learn about how helpful some other therapies can be. The body is, by far, the most interesting machine ever designed! When something is imbalanced, it acts like a constructive feedback system. It works in opposites by generating symptoms that are the result of problems in a very different area of the body. What this means is usually when there's a problem, it's not in the area you are feeling the pain. In addition, the actual problem areas usually "refer" the symptoms out through the fascial (spider web like structure running under the skin) and the nervous system (controls everything through the spinal column). Basically, every nerve has to go through your spine before it branches out to control your organs, muscles, and everything else. However, with a hard-working job you build up small subluxations (Luxation is Latin for broken, think "Sub Broken"). These block off the energy and electrical impulses that control everything.

The problem is, an estimated 80% of your nervous system is "non-sensory," meaning by the time you feel pain, the problem has already been there for some time. If most of these are not set up to feel pain, they have to find a way to call out to you. It's very common after some time for your body to slowly get sick and tired of you not listening to it, so it fights back and calls out to you with sometimes unexplainable symptoms to get your attention. Take a look at a picture of the spine and all of its vertebrae. See if you can trace the nerves from where you're feeling symptoms back to a specific vertebra area of the back. It may be that you need a chiropractic adjustment in that area to open things back up and restore normal energetic function to these areas. I have heard that some paramedics in Europe are being taught emergency chiropractic protocol in some cases when responding to a heart attack call. Is your heart going crazy because you need an alignment?

Your adjustment cannot be done just once! Muscle has memory, and it's likely the muscle will pull the subluxations (Spinal Knots) back into place unless you ease the tension and have a realignment every few weeks.

12
SAVING TIME & MONEY

Don't Guess, Assess

Some great assessments to use for identifying injuries, tracking progress, and creating a personal profile are listed below. If most of these aren't done when you start training, you should find a new gym.

- Nutrition and lifestyle assessment
- Body composition & metabolic-typing test
- Core strength & functional assessment
- 9-point flexibility test & postural analysis
- Blood pressure and resting heart rate test

By establishing your assessment profile, you can define your starting point and accurately measure your results week by week. This way, you know exactly where you are in relation to your goal and we can make any necessary adjustments as you progress, avoiding potential plateaus and injuries before they happen.

Educate Your Mind

You've heard it before: no two people are exactly the same. That's why a personalized program design is a science. This is where sound advice is unparalleled! Education in a "No-One-Size-Fits-All" approach is the keynote to your program, and trumps any book, video, or internet article you wish to try on your own. There are simply just too many variables to consider.

There are six essential components to maximize your results in minimal time:

- Nutrition
- Supplementation
- Resistance training
- Cardiovascular training
- Flexibility
- Accountability

Motivate Your Body

Most people think exercise and good nutrition has to hurt or taste bad to work. This cannot be farther from the truth! With all six of these components in place, you should lose 1.6 pounds of fat every week, while increasing lean muscle. A quality, successful personal trainer with your best interests in mind will create the accountability that you need to be successful in your program. Especially in the long term, looking past just one day.

Just knowing you can't "blow off your workout today" is half the battle. That's why external accountability to a coach makes such a huge difference.

Exercise Your Spirit

Getting the body you want won't be a "walk in the park." Nothing of lasting value is ever that easy. Exercise is where you take action with a personalized program, addressing every aspect of your nutrition and fitness as you move forward. Each session, we are assessing your mental, physical, and nutritional state before we get started. Bottom line: you need to have fun with your workouts. If it's not fun, you're not going to do it. Not many trainers know this, and that's what can give working out a bad name. Once you hit your goal, we can transition you to a maintenance program where things actually do get much easier.

Our personal training programs are world-class because they include both nutrition & fitness training, and are completely customized to your fitness goals and lifestyle. This means we spend a lot of time working with our clients on both the exercise AND the nutrition components that are required for getting serious results.

Big Gym Rip-Off

Well it should be obvious by this point: you're going to need a gym membership, or you're going to have to live in a cave and hunt for your food. Either way, we're going to need to get your activity levels up. Before you spend money anywhere, let's take a look at some of the biggest issues in commercial gym memberships. I know from personally working in this field that the name of the game was to sign up more people than are cancelling each day. This most certainly implies that most people that are paying for a gym membership are not using it. Most facilities will oversell their memberships because they know not everyone's going to show up.

This isn't to say that the people running the gym are evil. Just switch roles for a sec: when it comes to business, would you want to call up your members who weren't using their membership, advise them to cancel, and kill your cash flow? No way!

Now let's talk a little bit about how you'll pay for your services. You'll almost certainly need to fork over your bank information to the gym so they can start monthly billing. Just be careful. Some places have been known to randomly debit their clients for erroneous charges – charges so small, you question whether to even dispute them.

But what about missed payments? Now this is where it can get crazy. For example, if you miss a $25 payment and, because of gym policy, they add a $75 fee for missing your payment, you're sitting at $100 in debt. In 2 days (when the system tries to hit you for the cash again), congrats! You now owe the company $175 and, because of gym policy, automatically cancels your account (with an added $200 cancellation fee). Please make sure you are aware of exactly what the terms are so you know what you are getting into.

Some of these numbers might be a little bit of exaggeration, but the truth is that it's one of the main reasons even the largest gyms are going out of business.

Proper Setup Of A Health Club

I've studied many different types of gyms, wellness studios, and health clubs for years. This being said, I feel that my gym utilizes a method that works perfectly for both my clients and my trainers. Here's a breakdown:

The first thing people realize when they come in to Optymal is that we're a lot different than your average gym. We spend a lot of time working with our members on both the nutrition & fitness components that are required for getting you where you want to be.

We have some members that come in only for our classes and hold themselves accountable to their own workouts. On the other hand, we have some members that have full gym access and meet with us anywhere from 2-3 times per week. It just depends on their goals, motivation, and budget.

We all know nutrition & fitness assistance can be expensive, and let's face it: in this day and age, not many people can afford personal training 4 times each week. Putting that aside, how many could actually use it?

By having everyone work with a trainer, either one-on-one, or in a small group class they gain a support system. Here's the bottom line: having an accountability and support system is, by far, the most important thing when making lifelong changes to your personal health.

If you're in the area, pop by for a juice! I'll show you around the studio, print you off a clean-eating list, and help you get started on keeping a food journal.

We keep it simple! Getting the results you want is based on five key factors: food selection, caloric intake, sleep, stress, and activity level - all of which are covered by a simple and unique fitness formula.

Personally, I find it unacceptable that large gyms sell memberships for a year and continue to bill you even when you stop showing up about 3 months in. In my opinion, a health club & fitness studio should be set up so that you pay for what you use. The business model shouldn't be based around how many new contracts get signed, but based upon the progress and results of the clients. A good studio would also offer common programs such as Zumba, Pilates, and Hot Yoga. Some even offer more unique classes, like pole or belly dancing.

It's the structured environment of support, accountability and skilled guidance on nutrition, combined with expert training in effective, efficient, and exciting, metabolism-stoking exercise. Don't buy into the boring, dreadful, mind-numbing stuff you may be picturing in your head. We agree that it doesn't work because people just burn-out, get sick of it, and quit. What we do is fun and stimulating – because when you're getting real results, and real changes, almost instantly, and well, that's pretty motivating.

We went into this business not to become some nameless, faceless corporation full of fast-talking marketers and slick salespeople, but to revolutionize the health & fitness industry. We're a locally owned and operated small business completely committed to fulfilling the promises we make. Like you, I make my home here. This is my community, and I care about my neighbors.

Here, there's no "catch," or fine print. No clauses or gimmicks – none of that nonsense. You won't be badgered until you buy something. Your experience with us will be unlike any other you've ever had.

New Year's Revelations

Losing weight and getting in shape is one of the top three New Year's resolutions for a staggering majority of Canadians and Americans year-in and year-out. I think that's great! It's the follow-through that everyone struggles with. I know in the past I'd say to myself, "Ok, I'm going to start a juice fast, and I'm not going to eat any food at all, no meat and no starchy breads or pastas." Well, by day two, I'm short on time and I think to myself, "Well, an apple won't hurt and it's basically the same as me juicing it." By day four I'm saying, "Well, toast isn't an animal product and it's whole wheat." The rest is history.

A Johns Hopkins university study found that 93.8% of people drop this resolution before the end of January. Now this particular time of year makes it really hard for people to overcome the obstacles that stand in their way in achieving a real preeminent goal. Let's be honest, your schedule this time of year is usually so packed with family stuff, you often end up seeing the best of everyone's guilty pleasures. External accountability is the secret to getting it done during the hype this time of year. I found some great peer reviewed studies by the top experts on fitness, weight loss and behavior modification that really put it into perspective for you. Think about this before committing to a New Year's Resolution.

"Study participants experienced 100% better weight loss and fitness results, dropping pounds faster and keeping them off longer, when they teamed up with a buddy with whom they have an existing relationship." – Rena Wing, PhD behavioral scientist, Brown University, Founder, National Weight Control Registry

————

"Study participants reported significantly greater weight loss, health and fitness results when they had the support of family and friends." – Powers, T. A., Koestner, R., & Gorin, A. A. (2008). Families, Systems, & Health, 26(4), 404-416.

————

"Study participants who actively enlisted the social support of 3 or more friends experienced 176% greater long term success with their exercise and nutrition program than those who tried to do it on their own." – Wing, R. R., & Jeffery, R. W. (1999). Journal of Consulting and Clinical Psychology, 67(1), 132-138.

————

"Building a social support network can be THE determining factor (to your fitness and weight loss success). You need people who will hold you to your agreements." – St. John, B. (2003). Build a support SYSTEM. Shape Magazine, 22(6), 28

––––––––

"The participant's personal network provides invaluable social support for them in four ways: (1) it allows for empathy; (2) it ensures accountability to others; (3) it provides venting and advice seeking; and (4) it shares validation of the experience." – Sanford, A. (2010). Communication Studies, 61(5), 567-584.

––––––––

I'm sharing these studies with you for a very important reason. No one can be with you 24/7! You need to have an accountability mechanism built into your goal, like a nutrition journal or consistent communication with a coach or mentor. From what I have discovered, adding another layer of accountability and support makes an incredibly significant difference in the speed and certainty with which you permanently transform yourself. Accountability to yourself alone allows you to start rationalizing it away. Having some accountability to a spouse, partner, or friend is a great start, but they'll stop nagging you because they don't want to damage the relationship. It's not a question of self-discipline. Your achievements in life speak volumes about your discipline. It's not a question of time. The energy and revitalization that you will experience will give you more time by increasing your productivity. And it's not a question of cost either, because you could spend thousands on home fitness equipment, joining gyms, trying this diet and never getting the results you want.

In summary, the most common things I see people missing are (A) they don't have the knowledge to put together a complete program for themselves, (B) They don't have a workable plan of action that integrates both the nutrition and fitness components together, (C) They don't have the external accountability to get things done. In the end, it all boils down to external accountability! One of the biggest pitfalls people run into is what I call the "I Know" syndrome. Take a skinny guy who's complaining about being so skinny. You tell him he's got to lift heavier weights and eat more. What does he say? "I know, I know." If you need to lose weight, your doctor will tell you to start exercise more and eat less. What you end up saying is "I know, I know."

"I know, I know." is a mental shortcut that enables you to shut off your brain from taking the action you've learned with this book. Keep this in mind as you move forward. If you've room for improvement, maybe you really don't know. If you really knew, you'd probably be doing it already. And if you were doing it, you wouldn't need the Health Bible in the first place.

Fitness Competitions And Judgment Day

A challenge is something that will leave you stronger then when you started. It should be a little scary, because challenges will leave you with confidence after you're done. My first half marathon left me limping for a week and needing to take time off work. But, how easy was it for me to do 15 minutes of cardio after that? Simple! You want to find an event that will up your threshold for fitness and willingness to get it done. Don't think about it too hard. Just find something that seems impossible and sign yourself up for it right away. Take action!

Some of my favorite types of events involve raising money for a charity, by exercising for 30 minutes per day for 30 days with instruction, support, and personal training from a team you pulled together. The beauty of this is bringing other people into it with you. The popularity of shows like "The Biggest Loser" has created numerous fitness contests in cities everywhere. I personally love ones where, at the end of the contest, people are awarded a grand prize, or where the winner may choose to have the $500 donated to a charity of their choice. My club gives to charities all the time and we are starting to host more and more of these types of competitions. There's something really powerful about the way you feel about yourself when you finish a fitness challenge. It's the feeling of real ownership of your life and passion for living it. You get in touch with yourself, your family, your goals and dreams in a way that just can't be conveyed in words – it has to be experienced.

What is sad is the fear that is holding so many people back from experiencing just that. Women in particular, are afraid of failing because there is so much pressure on them. Especially if they've tried to lose weight or get in shape before and have not been successful. Over time, that kind of thing can really undermine your confidence. Here's what is really interesting: losing weight and getting in great shape is not nearly as difficult as you may think when you have the right kind of help. In fact, few things have been studied and analyzed as much as the science behind weight loss and fitness.

Getting the kind of results you can see in the mirror and feel when you put on your clothes can be accomplished in a reasonably short period of time when you're all-in for a fitness event, regardless of where you are physically right now. The weight loss industry, the pharmaceutical industry, the diet industry, and the pre-packaged food companies like Jenny Craig and NutriSystem all want you to believe their secrets are the best. These secrets always involve buying their food, their pills, their gizmo, gadget, or whatever. People need to be in a structured environment that provides emotional support, consistency and accountability. It's a bit like school! You need the structure in the early stages so you can quickly learn how to think and perform like the pros you see in the ads for these events and competitions. Most people never get the structure they need when it comes to their health and fitness. So, the natural tendency is to hope the shortcuts and "magic bullets" will work. As anyone who's tried them can tell you, there's no magic in those bullets.

No Gym Equipment – No Problem

Too often, we use the excuse that because we can't get to the gym, we can't get in shape. It's time we put a stop to all of that. That's why I wrote this section: to save you from yourself -and guess what? You're not going to need any expensive equipment for any of these exercises. To top it all off, you really won't need much space either.

The trick is to make exercise a habit and that's easy to do with these exercises. They're simple, fast, and super effective. I have even put together a schedule for you, so just pick dates and you're ready to rock! Get started by doing the following exercises and you'll be seeing some results, fast. I've trained lots of trainers, so I guess you can say that I know what I'm talking about. At my facility we're not just about getting you some protein powder and a typical exercise regimen then sending you on your way. Enough about us, let's talk about you the Primal Patterns movements: and the 6 best anytime, anywhere exercises that you don't even know you already use!

What Are The Primal Patterns?

Primal Patterns movements are based on the physiology of how the body moves. Basically, we've been designed through millions of years of evolution to move a certain way in order to survive as a species. When you break it down, every movement the human body is capable of doing can be reduced to only 6 movements. They are as follows:

Push – Pushing doors open, shoveling snow.

Pull – Pulling doors open, taking something off a shelf.

Twist – Getting in and out of your car.

Squat – Going to the washroom.

Lunge – Walking up stairs, advancing from crawling to walking.

Bend – Picking something up, tying your shoes.

When you look around at a gym that is filled with machines or reflect on exercises you've done in the past, you can break them down into one or more of the six movements. Once you understand this, all of the exercises you've ever heard of start to make sense. This is called functional exercise. Bottom line: you should never exercise on machines!

Why Does This Matter To Me?

Let's face it, not everyone wants to exercise just to look good. Anyone who's ever incurred previous injury or pain induced from exercise understands how important it is to move properly, not just in the gym, but during all day-to-day activities. Having a weak core is like driving a car with wheels that aren't aligned. Granted you can make it to work and back, but good luck getting that puppy to take you across the country. Train your core to support your body through your exercises and daily life. Get off the machines! Work your core, every rep!

Primal Pattern One: The Push

Yeah, you guessed it, I'm talking about push-ups! I know most people dread doing push-ups, and that's a shame because it's the "ultimate exercise." Once you get into the habit of doing them, they're a cinch! While you're doing those push-ups, you're working your arms, chest, core, and legs! If you can spend just 5-10 minutes per day doing push-ups, you'll see and feel amazing results in a very short period of time. Best of all, you can do them anywhere and there's no need for any bulky, expensive gym equipment.

Here's how to do a proper, crisp, and sexy push-up!

1. Get comfy, and lie face down on the floor.
2. Put your palms on the floor, just about level with your breast and fairly tight to your body.
3. Now's the time to push up. Make sure you keep the rest of your body rigid.
4. Stop pushing up just before you lock your elbows. Hold that for a second and then lower yourself back down slowly, until your nose is almost touching the floor.
5. That's one! Now lather, rinse and repeat.

Primal Pattern Two: The Pull

Here you'll see how to do a row. This is another great anywhere, anytime exercise. All you need is something small that weighs over 5 pounds. Rows are an excellent pulling exercise. Although they're especially good at working and toning your back, if you're trying to lose the flab on the back of your arms, a daily round of rows should help it disappear.

So here's how to do it!

1. Stand to the right of a bench with a weight/object in your right hand.
2. With your left knee on the bench, let your right arm hang down and forward a bit.
3. Tighten up those abs and arch your back.

4. Bend forward at the hips keeping your back parallel to the floor.
5. Slightly bend your right knee and tilt your chin toward your chest.
6. Pull your right arm up, point your elbow at the ceiling, until your hand comes up to your rib cage.
7. Slowly lower the weight back down.
8. Repeat on both sides.

Primal Pattern Three: The Twist

Well, I think you know what's coming, if not, you can definitely smell it cooking. The Standing Russian Twist! It's important you keep your hands on the ball in front of your chest. A standing Russian twist targets the oblique muscles through rotation of the spine. The abs are also getting some love while they support the spine throughout this exercise. This is a great all-around exercise that really helps to build endurance throughout your entire core. Talk about a rock-solid foundation for success!

Here's how to do a twist!

1. Stand with your feet shoulder-width apart and hold a medicine ball with your arms straight in front of your abdomen.
2. Twist to the left and then twist to the right and push the ball to the wall.
3. Repeat.

Primal Pattern Four: The Lunge

Don't worry about looking strange here, you're just getting back in touch with your primal side. You can do this in the privacy of your own home and it's more than excellent for toning your legs. Lunges will strengthen your legs, knees, and help you develop better posture, balance, and stability. Because you're working large muscles, you'll burn off more calories too. Still, put down the cheeseburger. Hold weights or water bottles for an even better, more intense, workout.

Here's how to do a lunge!

1. Take a big stride forward.
2. Bend your back leg so your knee just about touches the floor.
3. Your front leg will also bend at the knee.
4. Now simply walk forward, bending your legs like this. Keep your upper body straight and rigid, it's all about good form.
5. Repeat.

Primal Pattern Five: The Squat

Like the push-up, this is an exercise you'll either love or hate. However, it's also incredibly beneficial to your health. You just need to make it a habit. It's important to keep your back straight as you squat. Squatting is great for adding strength to your legs and working your core too.

Here's how to pop a squat!

1. Stand up with your arms by your side. Feet about one foot apart.
2. Now sink your butt to the floor, bending at the knees.
3. As you go down pull your arms up, so they're straight out in front of you.
4. When you go down as far as you can, hold for a second.
5. Now use your legs to stand up straight again, moving your arms back to the side of your body.
6. Repeat.

Primal Pattern Six: The Dead-Lift

There's no better compound exercise that targets the quads, hamstrings, gluteal muscles, lower back, and forearms like the dead-lift. It's important to keep your back straight as you lift. Bending is great for adding strength to your legs and working your core too.

Here's how to do a dead-lift!

1. Grab something that has some dead weight to it and step up to it.
2. Keep your feet shoulder width apart.
3. From your hips, tilt your back towards the floor.
4. Before your back becomes parallel to the floor, bend your knees while keeping your back straight to get closer to the ground.
5. Look straight ahead.

6. Lift the weight by raising your hips and shoulders at the same time and speed while keeping your abs tight.
7. Come to a standing position with your shoulders pulled back, allowing the weight to hang in front of your hips.
8. Return the weight to its starting position in a clean, controlled manner, while squeezing your glutes and keeping your head up.
9. Repeat

Your Running-Start Exercise Plan

Week: _____

Exercise Time Reps
Push-Up 5 minutes
Row 5 minutes
Russian Twist 5 minutes
Lunge 5 minutes
Squat 5 minutes
Bend 5 minutes

___Day 01 ___Day 02 ___Day 03

Instructions

Print this page every week and stick it on your fridge, your toilet, by your computer, or somewhere else where you'll see it often. Fill out your own reps. The goal here is to increase them over the next few months. Start at around 20-40 (depending on how fit you feel you are) and then raise the bar every couple of weeks. Do this 3 times a week. Check off Day 01, Day 02 and Day 03 after you complete each day. It's good to set out specific days to help form the habit. For example, block in your calendar for Monday, Wednesday and Friday. Don't forget to take five minutes before and after for warm-up and cooldown.

Avoiding Plateaus

You may be surprised to hear this, but taking an active recovery week every few months by relaxing your goals and behaviors is healthy from time to time. Periodization is a program model trainers use based on changing your workouts and meals over time to achieve different results and to keep you from plateauing. Its structure looks like this, in a nutshell:

Foundation: Normally high rep exercises with a focus on learning form.

Strength: Generally reps of 8-12 to build strength needed for the next phase.

Burn: Low rest periods during workouts with lots of reps and sets.

Power: Usually weights that are more challenging for you. Low reps with high weight to spark new muscle fibers.

Your first training phase after your foundation might be devoted to getting stronger, while the next phase might be devoted to getting leaner. In between these phases, I always encourage an active recovery week or vacation. What works for exercise can also work for diet as well. Instead of killing yourself by pursuing hard-core fat loss for the next year straight, why not break down your commitment into phases?

This is a much better approach, both psychologically and physiologically. The beauty is that you can plan your nutritional commitment around big events, holidays, and summer BBQs. Let's say you travel extensively in June and July. Well, why not ramp up your commitment during the spring so that during the summer you can relax a bit? Break down your commitment over the next year. If you fail to plan, you plan to fail. Decide what your commitment level is (I have based it on three levels and it's always worked for me). Figure out how many meals are required at each level. Then print off a calendar of the year ahead and plan your nutritional commitment around these events, based on these levels.

Extremely Committed: 42 healthy meals & snacks per week, with lots of water during and after meals.

Committed: Having less than 42 healthy meals & snacks per week, with lots of water.

Not Committed: Consuming only 21 healthy meals & snacks per week, with lots of water.

What To Take From This

All these exercises are classic, time-tested proven winners – just like you! Now it's time for the hard part, the commitment. Print off your weekly schedule. Stick to it religiously for about 1 month (that's it, baby!), and you'll begin to make a habit out of working out. That's the goal! Commit to these goals and you'll have a healthier body that looks better naked.

13
MENTALLY & PHYSICALLY FIT

If not being able to get to the gym has been holding you back from the body you deserve, these "mental exercises" will fix you up. You need absolutely no special equipment for them, just a little bit of time. The exercises in this chapter are, by far, some of the most powerful you will ever find. Try reading through the sections and practicing the exercises for a few days and amazing things will happen!

Most people today are trying numerous approaches to look and feel better, but they are often just spinning their wheels. The fact that you are reading this chapter already sets you apart from the "others." Sit back, relax and allow me to explain some naturally complex subjects in a language that you can understand.

Get started by learning the exercises below in order and, in no time, you will see amazing results, sure-fire and fast! As a premier health and fitness expert, I have coached tons of clients to amazing body transformations, so you know everything I am about to share is proven. Not just with them, but with myself as well. Everyone, somewhere in the course of their program, runs into a wall and has to start to implement the concepts discussed in this chapter.

A Typical Day

You've been so busy trying to maintain your social life and prepare for tomorrow's workday that you've totally lost track of time. It's almost midnight and you're reconsidering your meal choices or lack thereof that day. Plus, you didn't get a chance to work out, so you know you're going to feel a bit lazy tomorrow. At least you can wind down and watch some television before bed. After a quick trip to the bathroom you realize you can't sleep because tomorrow's busy schedule is racing through your mind. The next thing you know the snooze button is calling you and you can't believe it's morning already. Your eyes were just ready to close. You head for the kitchen searching for coffee, waking the children and grabbing your cell. As you go through the motions, your brain is trying to figure out how to get everything done before you leave the house. Finally, you're ready to go when you realize you haven't eaten anything again.

Work is crazy, as usual, and by lunch you're running to grab something nice and "preserved" to eat, or maybe another cup of coffee will do. You realize you won't have time to exercise today, and you forgot to pay that bill again. Then someone calls you and reminds you of that social event to which you committed the other day. By five, you're racing to the grocery store to try and pick up some healthy foods for dinner.

Seeing as how you didn't settle for Lean Cuisine again, the result is a pile of dishes and you're exhausted! At least you have a nice vacation coming up for which to prepare. You can start exercising next week, once things calm down.

Most people spend way too much time focusing on physical things and the world around them that they forget what really matters. When you do this you lack the power to maximize your mental capacity and neglect the spiritual you.

Here's the bottom line: exercising for the wrong reason and without a positive mindset will get you nowhere! Remember, your emotional and mental state manifests itself physically within the body, your thoughts, your posture and mostly the choices you make. Consider where you may be out of balance. Good things come in threes: like your mind, body, and spirit. You want to be balanced to get real results from any program. Start making that mind-body-spirit connection, balance yourself in the direction that's needed, and get that peace of mind!

Mental Exercises

Your personal success in life is directly connected to the quality and quantity of questions you ask on a daily basis. With this in mind, most of us live our lives unwilling to ask questions, either in fear of being viewed as stupid, or because of a lack of interest in new things. As we have all heard, the only stupid question is the one not asked, especially with regard to physical exercise. Asking quality questions should be the first step towards manifesting what you want in your physical life.

Directed positive thought is the keynote to getting fitness results, as each thought has an immensely powerful energy. Knowing this, you can implement concentrated mental energy to free yourself from negative thought patterns. In doing so, you will enhance your self-confidence, become more grounded, and enjoy a much more productive life. At first, simply listen to your "self-talk." Do you often start a sentence with "I don't," or, "I can't," or, "I probably won't?" If you analyze the thought messages that are being conveyed with these words, you'll know exactly why you never have any real fitness results. Shifting old patterns can be hard work. But don't give up; you will be rewarded!

If you "bad mouth" someone, that particular negative energy will come back to you. It's karma! Everyone has something unique to offer, so use your newfound insight to identify each person's good qualities. Don't be drawn into negative conversations. If a friend regularly becomes involved in disastrous situations, be empathetic and then ask them what he or she can learn from that pattern to prevent the same thing from happening again.

Although positive thought has many benefits, it can't be used as a solution for illness. It should never be used as a way of hiding or denying pain. If you have a problem, confront it, and then use effective affirmations to change any damaging, fixed patterns of behaviour. Once you have learned to harness the power of positive thought, you'll find yourself stair-stepping your life towards success. Use this extraordinary technique to improve every aspect of your life, to help you get a better job, to improve your talents, or to bring you radiant good health.

Health: "My body is the temple of my soul and looks after me perfectly"

Courage: "I am one with the universe and safe at all times"

Employment: "Perfect work for perfect pay is coming my way"

Love: "I love the world and it loves me"

Success: "Abundance and success now come to me in endless ways"

Happiness: "I am balanced, joyful, happy and radiant and detached from any fear"

Prosperity: "The universe is an endless source which pours wealth upon me"

What Is Stress?

Stress is very often the root of many people's problems, whether they realize it or not. You may feel overstressed now or you may not even realize that you are stressed because you have grown used to it day by day. Understanding what exactly stress does to the body and the different forms it comes in will help you make better decisions and completely change your life!

You probably think of stress as bad, but that isn't always the case. Just as bones and muscles need exercise to stay strong, we also need certain amounts of stress to stay healthy. A complete lack of stress would not be a good thing; its keeps your thinking sharp both consciously and subconsciously.

There are six major types of stress; each has good and bad effects. Try to identify which types are affecting you most, then try doing things differently to balance out the effects of stress.

Physical Stress – vigorous exercise or a labour-intensive job.

Nutritional Stress – eating too much, too little, or preserved foods.

Mental Stress – "stinking thinking", over-studying, taking on too much.

Chemical Stress – caffeine, pesticides, herbicides, fungicides and a few fertilizers.

Electronic Stress – electronic devices, cell phones, computers, treadmills, TV.

Thermal Stress – body temperature: being "too hot" or "too cold" for too long.

Stress Reduction

Failing to reduce your stress is the #1 thing that will sabotage all of your health and fitness goals. The faster you realize this, the faster you will get results. Your body doesn't know the difference between good and bad stress. Whether or not you are getting married or have lost someone close to you, the physiological responses are the same to the body. When you start to take on more physical exercise, it is imperative to understand that stress reduction will play a key role in the results you want. If you can identify the difference between physical and mental stressors, you can learn to balance them and empower your results tenfold!

There are hundreds of self-help books and many concepts to reducing stress. Allow me to strongly recommend these simple methods, which are hands down the simplest to use and the best that I have found. They are tried, tested, and true ways to a "stress-less" lifestyle that I teach to all my clients all the time. The following takes only minutes a day, guarantees you results and will totally supercharge your day by attracting the positive things you want. If you can relate to the 'typical day" as mentioned in the introduction, then these three simple steps will help you begin to move in the right direction.

Step 1 - Power Up in the Morning: 1-5 Minutes
Starting your morning in a "fight or flight" mode by waking the children, text messaging and worrying about the day is the reason why you are making unhealthy choices and not working out as consistently as you need. Honestly, how you start your day dictates everything that

follows. Instead of going right to your normal routine take five minutes to get yourself into a relaxed, meditative state and find an inspirational statement that you can affirm to promote your well-being for that day. The key here is to totally clear your head and take in the bigger picture. Realize that you are not running the show and that there is more to this world than you. Use some of the following guidelines to find a way that works best for you. Keep it simple – simply clearing your head can be hard enough sometimes, start here.

Be inventive – Randomly open a book and find a word you want to reflect on that day.

Catchphrase – convert it into a memorable rhyme – no more than four lines.

Affirmation – Say it out loud at least three times a day, for at least 21 days.

Write It Out – If you don't write it down on paper you are not making it real.

Step 2 - Activate into Exercise

Now get out a pen and paper and "write out" what you are going to do for exercise that day. Then plan when you will be going to unwind later on in the evening. Remember if you don't write it out you won't make it real and it simply won't happen! A study done years ago with Harvard graduates showed time and time again; those who write out their goals, achieve them, and it only takes a few seconds. Not to mention this is the theme from the first chapter. Whatever positive thought or catchphrase you write out will sub-consciously change the decisions you make and the course of your day. Write out what exactly you are going to commit to that day for healthy activity. This could be a walk, workout or just taking the stairs for a change.

Step 3 - Unwind in the Evenings: 10-15 Minutes

At the end of the day you have carried home with you the day's stressors and you probably don't even realize it. In order to let go of them, you have to unwind before you play the spouse or parent role with your family. Think of it as "you time" where you are dropping off all the mental baggage you brought home with you. The main focus is to quiet your mind so that you can reduce the harmful bodily effects that stress causes. The most common effects are poor sleep and zero results from your new fitness program. Plus, you just simply become a better person. Use some of the following guidelines to find a way that works best for you:

Go Outside – A slow walk with the dog while noticing your natural surroundings. Take in the bigger picture, look at the clouds or sky.

Shower/Bath – Warm water can be very relaxing and good for the body. Add in some Epson's salts, turn off the lights and light a few candles.

Meditate – Quit your mind by stopping at a coffee shop or waiting in the driveway before heading into the house.

Sex – If lack of communication is a problem, unwind and unleash. Sex is the most communicative act we have.

Did You Say Meditation

If you have a stressful life, or do any form of rigorous physical activity, an important skill is being able to calm your mind and body. This will enhance your ability to rest properly, make better choices, learn more and have the mind-body connections necessary to create the life you really want. Meditation is the best way to do this! If you've never meditated before you may think it's for crazy yoga instructors or Chinese wizards. However, it is simply a pleasant way of escaping from the stressors of the day. This state of mind is precisely what you need to achieve the mind-body connection that improves your life so dramatically. Once you realize it, you will always make time for it.

Meditation sharpens and focuses your mental activity and keeps you alert at work, at home and in your relationships. Most of the physical exercises you do should involve some quality focus and proper breathing. The following techniques are some of the most effective ways of doing this. Once you have become completely familiar with meditation, you'll have the key to opening yourself up to a new world of experiences. In this way, meditation can dramatically change your life.

Guidelines To Meditation

1. Find a clean, quiet, airy, comfortable, uncluttered place and dedicate this spot to relaxation – meditating in the same area builds up a positive energy.

2. Turn off your phone before starting and lock the door if you think you might be disturbed.

3. Wear comfortable, loose, clean clothing. Consider a bath, shower or at least wash your hands.

4. You may want to use something to focus your meditation' this can be an object such as a candle, flower, or picture, a sound such as a mantra or ambient music can help.

5. Sit in a chair or on the floor with your back supported. Place your arms on your legs with your hands in an open position – this puts you in the right posture.

6. Devote your whole attention to your point of focus; start with five minutes then gradually increase the time to twenty if possible.

7. Do not force your mind to concentrate! Keep it focused, but without effort. When thoughts intrude, don't push them away, but let them float by. If your mind wanders, return it to its focus, no matter how often it escapes.

8. It's a good idea to meditate at the same time of day – many people choose first thing in the morning, as meditation is usually better on an empty stomach. Meditation at night can help you let go of all the day's stressors. Find a time that suits you to meditate regularly.

You may need to explore several avenues before you discover the approach to meditation that works best for you. Each of the pathways described ahead offers a slightly different focus, and some may work better for you in the beginning. None are "better" than others – they are simply alternatives. Whatever route you choose, you'll intuitively know when you've arrived at that calm place. This is the point of meditation.

Aids To Meditation

Music – You may find that special meditative music tapes or certain classical pieces can help to clear the mind of intrusive thoughts. If you have never meditated before, music may be just what you need to help you in the beginning.

Mantra – The repetition of a single sound, word, or phase produces a powerful force that will block the intrusion of other thoughts. You may wish to focus on personally meaningful word. You can say it aloud or repeat it silently. It can be helpful to synchronize your mantra with your breathing, saying it on every out or in breath. If your attention wanders, gently bring it back to your mantra.

Light – A lit candle placed in front of you can help work as a point of focus if you prefer to meditate with your eyes open. First close your eyes then breathe deeply in and out through your nose. Slowly open your eyes and gaze at the flame.

Objects – The visual stimulus of a simple object like a leaf, shell, candle, flower, or petal can help to concentrate your mind during meditation. So too can a pleasant fragrance such as incense. Always use what works for you, these are just a few suggestions.

Breath – Breathing is the simplest of focus and when you observe its natural rhythms it can help to calm the mind. Let each breath enter and leave your body at its normal pace. Observe how your chest moves with the rest of your body even though you are still. If you'd like, you can count the inhalations and exhalations to help you stay focused. Inhale to the count of 4, and then exhale to the count of 4.

Proper Breathing

Breathing properly is the key to every exercise and all relaxation techniques. Most people breathe improperly by taking shallow breaths. If you have ever watched young children play sports, their tummies move in and out because they are using all the respiratory muscles properly to draw air into the deepest part of the lungs. Deep, proper breathing is also the way to take your meditation to the next level. This exercise is easy and the key to complete relaxation; it can last as long or as short of a time as you wish.

Work in a quiet room where you feel relaxed. You may want to put on some soothing music to help you wind down. When you are completely calm, turn off the music and concentrate.

Direct your conscious awareness onto your breathing or just the sound of your breath alone.

Tune into the "ebb and flow" of your breath and gently focus onto its quiet rhythm so that everything is at one with your breathing. Take your time while doing this – you are entering a deep meditative state.

Let your breath take you to your inner "calm place" and consciously visualize breathing out tension and breathing in the feeling of relaxation.

Visualize your breathing as ripples moving outward from your body in increasingly larger circles, or as waves of energy radiating from your body.

Deliberately hold the energy and keep your focus – don't be tempted to feel frustrated if it isn't working as well as you'd like. After a while, as you breathe, concentrate on the thought that every living thing breathes in energy. Say to yourself "we all breathe in energy." Now let yourself become completely open to the universal forces of energy. Stay with this feeling as long as you like.

When you're ready, gently lead your consciousness back into your physical body, paying particular attention to keeping your feet on the ground. Finally, cross your arms and legs as an act of closing.

Fine-Tuning Your Focus

In the Eastern part of the world, concepts of vitality and health are much different. If you look at a colour spectrum, you'll notice that each colour vibrates at a different frequency. The body has different centres of spinning energy sometimes seen as radiant colours at seven points along the spinal column. These are called chakras.

Each one of these colours has a specific physical, emotional, and mental correspondent and is the basis of most alternative therapies such as yoga, acupuncture, and many others. The chakra centres are an important part of the picture because visualizing colour can act as a focal point for meditation. As described, each chakra radiates the energy of its colour, starting from the top of the body. These are violet, indigo, blue, green, yellow, orange, and red. They represent how you interact with the world and experience yourself.

The breathing exercise earlier is an excellent starting point. You can use the visualization of colour exercise below to check for any problems in your chakras or energy levels. This should be fun and experimental, not complex and frustrating. Give it a chance; you might impress yourself with what you find.

An Experimental Journey

There is no right or wrong way to do this exercise. It will help free your mind and identify some interesting things you didn't notice about your life. Focus your mind onto your chakras and let yourself be intuitively drawn towards one of them. Now, visualize a door in front of you that is the signature colour of that chakra. See yourself move towards the door, step by step, and open the door slowly.

Visualize yourself opening the door and then entering the room beyond.

Now Consider These Questions

- What does the room look like?
- What is on the walls?
- What furniture is in the room?
- Is there a closet or drawers? If so, what is inside?
- Is there a picture on the wall? If so, describe it.
- How does the room feel generally?
- Is anyone else in the room? What is he or she communicating?
- How reluctant are you to leave the room?

What To Take From This

Interpreting what you see can be made very complex however there are some basic things to consider. The way you feel about this room relates to the energy of the chakra you chose. You will have to do some research to figure out what you are dealing with. If you see colours that are strong, vibrant and clear, that's fine; but if they are dark or muddy you have a few problems to resolve. Furniture represents burdens and anything found in drawers or closets relates to what you need to discard. Also, any pictures on the walls are an image of you. The healthiest state of the room is completely empty. If your room is cluttered, you have a lot of unfinished business connected with the area of yourself that you are exploring here.

14

FOCUS ON HEALTH NOT WEALTH

I've tried everything known to man to get results for myself and my clients. The one thing I can say is this: no matter what it is, you get what you pay for. It's not enough to live life halfway! You can make your life better! I don't want to sound shallow but, you know in your heart that if you lose some body fat and tone up a bit, you will be happier, healthier, and more self-confident.

I can show you an honest, simple, reliable, legitimate, and fast fat loss and fitness system that can do it for you! I am not trying to "sell" you anything, but I do have a powerful solution. It's a 10-week program based on years of trial and error, years of study, and years of real-life application. You'll have to engage in a moderate exercise program and eat a more healthy diet in order to safely, effectively, and rapidly lose body fat and keep it off permanently!

There is no "miracle" fat loss program out there. You may not believe it now, but losing fat and getting fit is not as difficult as you think. Anyone can enjoy a lean, toned body if they just understand the basic, fundamental principles I've discussed in the Health Bible, and then apply them to their daily life.

But keep an open mind that no matter how hard you work, if the underlying system is weak, you'll never achieve the permanent fat loss you're looking for. That's why I encourage you to investigate my program, a system that is time-tested and proven! One second, is this a sales pitch? Right now you are probably saying to yourself, "Rob said he wasn't going to try to sell me anything, and this is beginning to sound suspiciously like a sales pitch!"

Remember how I said I would reveal the truth to you about the deceptive practices of the nutrition and fitness industries? I can confidently say that I gave you really valuable information about the lies that are being fed to you. Plus, I gave you valuable information about what you can do to empower yourself against this misinformation. I don't think that alone addresses the problems you face. There really is so much to learn and, generally we all learn by doing. I think it would be careless if I didn't share a proven system for achieving your fat loss and goals. It would be like telling you there's a cure for cancer, but not telling you what it is!

Well, I want to give you the cure! I will say it again, I'm not trying to convince you of anything you don't want to do. Most people can't be "sold," anyway. We naturally throw up barriers when we think someone's trying to "sell" us something. All of my processes are to educate and inform. Nothing more! What you do with this information is your business. My hope is you will take action and pass this book along to a family member.

ABOUT THE AUTHOR

Rob believes that what others say about you as a group conscience is most times, your best judge of character. As a certified personal trainer and nutritionist, his approach is very holistic in nature, and helpful for the average person he sees as being stuck on autopilot - which he has proved time and time again with countless testimonials to his name. Aside from his list of high profile clients, what fuels his passion is bringing average people to above average standards.

He is the senior trainer and owner of Optymal Health Studios, located in the heart of downtown Whitby. His entrepreneurial spirit, juice cleansing programs and Hot Yoga studio speak volumes about his approach to health and fitness. He currently holds the voted title as Durham Region's Best Personal Trainer by the Durham Business Times Magazine, and is a contributing health and fitness writer for SNAP Newspaper.

When Rob is not juice bar tending, he can be found public speaking about mental and physical health throughout his community and at local schools. He believes that personal trainers and nutritionists are a dime a dozen and shouldn't be trusted if they only have testimonials, or a "cheesy" sounding money back guarantee. With the launch of his new book and line of supplements, he strives to help more people discover a happier healthier lifestyle, one day at a time!

Field Notes

Dirty Little Secrets

Hello good friend!

I wanted to personally thank you for picking up my book. I was told not to call it "The Health Bible" because some people may feel like I have offend their beliefs. When, In fact, the opposite is true! My goal is <u>to capture those with an open mind</u> and save them from years of going up and down in body fat, meal after meal, year after year, relationship after relationship.

My philosophy is that a structured nutrition and fitness program is useless unless you are self-aware enough to see where you are "dropping the ball" on taking action. So... to bridge that gap, my gift to you is a <u>complementary personal training session</u>. Its not Frankincense and Mur I know, but it's the least I could do for a potential friend.

I'm on my own journey just as you are. If chatting about nutrition and fitness strategy will help you out, it would be my pleasure to connect. <u>Real, lasting, positive change only comes from within</u>, and I'm positive I can help you do that no matter what your situation is. I've done it before with hundreds of others.

You can bring a friend or family member if you like, I'm totally cool with that! I'll roll out the red carpet, <u>make you a juice on the house,</u> and hook you up with a food journal before you leave.

Yours truly,

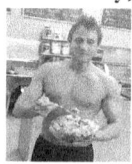

Author of The Health Bible
(905) 556-2202
rob@optymalhealthstudios.com

P.S. – <u>Don't spend any money on health programs</u> until you come see me. At least give yourself something to compare it to. Nobody wants average anymore.

P.S.S. – Check out our Optymal Health Studios Facebook page, the <u>best judge of character is what others think as a group conscious.</u>

www.ingramcontent.com/pod-product-compliance
Lightning Source LLC
Chambersburg PA
CBHW060503290526
45791CB00001B/252